The Art and Science
of
Burn Wound Management

The Art and Science of Burn Wound Management

Marella L Hanumadass MD
Former Chairman, Division of Burn Surgery and
Former Director, Sumner L.Koch Burn Center
Cook County Hospital
Chicago, Illinois, USA

and

K Mathangi Ramakrishnan
MB FRCS (Eng) FRCS (Edin) MCh (Plastic) DSc FAMS
Chief of Burn and Plastic Surgery
KK CHILDS Trust Hospital, Chennai
Emeritus Professor of Plastic Surgery
Tamil Nadu Dr MGR Medical University
Chennai, Tamil Nadu, India

With Special Contribution by

Mary Babu PhD
Department of Biotechnology
Central Leather Research Institute
Adyar, Chennai, Tamil Nadu, India

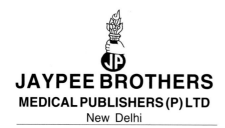

JAYPEE BROTHERS
MEDICAL PUBLISHERS (P) LTD
New Delhi

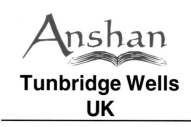

**Tunbridge Wells
UK**

First published in the UK by

Anshan Ltd
in 2005
6 Newlands Road
Tunbridge Wells
Kent TN4 9AT, UK

Tel/Fax: +44 (0)1892 557767
E-mail: info@anshan.co.uk
www.anshan.co.uk

ISBN 1 904798 365

British Library Cataloguing in Publication Data
A catalogue record for this book is available from the British Library

Printed in India by Gopsons Papers Ltd., A-14, Sector 60,Noida

Preface

"Medicine is a science of uncertainty and an art of probability."

Sir William Osler

Management of burn injuries, like many other medical disciplines, is still a developing science. However, in the western world and especially in the last three decades, there has been a remarkable decrease in the incidence of major burns, associated mortality and an improved quality of life of burn victims. Yet during this same period, although great strides have been made, the incidence and mortality rate remain very high in India and Southeast Asia. Realizing the need for a comprehensive treatise on this subject to cater to the needs of physicians practicing in the subcontinent, we published "Handbook of Burns Management" in 1990. Accomplished burn surgeons from both India and the United States of America contributed various chapters.

In the past decade, most of the progress in burns care has been in our better understanding of the pathophysiology of the burn wound and development of innovative methods of wound management. Our current work "The Art and Science of Burn Wound Management" is dedicated to this aspect of burns care.

Several disciplines contribute to the successful outcome of a patient with major burns. However, it is important to keep in mind that healing of the wound alone is not the end point. In that respect, our work like the previous one is not a complete treatise on the subject, but is confined to the medical and surgical aspects of burn wound management. We highlight the basic aspects of burn wound management as well as the recent advances in pathophysiology and clinical management. Early wound closure, biological dressings and skin substitutes developed in India and the United States of America are covered in great detail. Procedures that are now only of historical importance and limited application, such as subescharclysis with antibiotics or enzymatic debridement of burn wounds are completely omitted. All the chapters are illustrated with color photographs for greater clarity and understanding.

Our thanks to Dr. Mary Babu for her help and special contribution to the chapter on Pharmacological Modulation of the Burn Wound.

We are grateful to Jaypee Brothers Medical Publishers who encouraged us to undertake this project.

This manual is intended as a practical guide for the clinician. We hope it will stimulate the laboratory scientist to unravel new ways of managing burn injuries.

Marella L Hanumadass
K Mathangi Ramakrishnan

Acknowledgements

We would like to express our appreciation to all the patients whom we had the privilege of treating at Sumner L. Koch Burn Center at Cook County Hospital, Chicago, USA, the burn care facility at Kilpauk Medical College Hospital and the KK Child's Trust Hospital, Chennai, India. Studying the progression and outcome of our patients inspired the publication of *The Art and Science of Burn Wound Management*.

We would also like to thank Dr V Jayaraman, Assistant Professor in the Department of Burns, Plastic and Reconstructive Surgery at Kilpauk Medical College, Chennai, for his tireless help in the preparation of this manuscript.

Marella L Hanumadass
K Mathangi Ramakrishnan

Contents

PART I
Basic Sciences

Anatomy of the Burn Wound

NORMAL STRUCTURE OF THE HUMAN SKIN

The skin is the largest bilayer organ in the human body. It is a tough, supple layer that covers the entire surface of the body. For an average adult, the skin surface area is approximately 3,000 square inches (7,500 centimeters). The thickness of the skin increases gradually after birth until about the age of 40 and then slowly begins to thin down. The skin provides a protective coverage for the internal structures and organs and performs a variety of functions that are essential for sustenance of life **(Figure 1.1A)**.

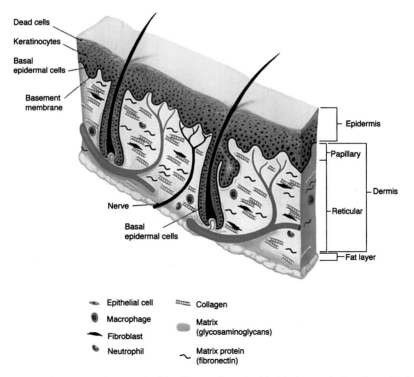

Figure 1.1A: Anatomy of normal skin (*Reproduced* with kind permission from Robert H Demling, MD from his monogram, 'partial-thickness burns current concepts as to pathogenesis and treatment').

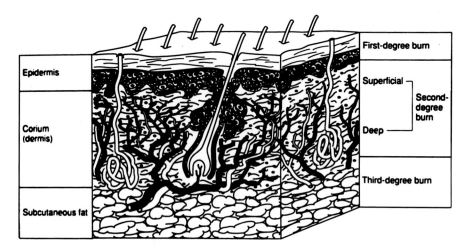

Figure 1.1B: Cross-section of the skin showing the layers of skin, skin appendages and depths of burn injury. (Reproduced with kind permission from WB Saunders Company: JAJ Martyn, MD. "Acute Management of Burned Patient," 1990 Edition, Page 13, Figure 2-1)

The principal structure of the skin consists of two layers: the outer thinner layer known as the *epidermis* which is composed of stratified squamous epithelium organized in five layers of strata and is avascular. The epidermis varies in thickness from 0.04 mm on the eyelids to 1.6 mm on the palms, with an average thickness of less than 0.17 mm ($^1/_{200th}$ of an inch) in most areas, except for those areas chronically exposed to pressure and friction.

Stratum Corneum

In this the outer most cells that contain the tough protein keratin are known as keratinocytes. They consist of 25-30 rows of dead flat, cells. The cells are continuously shed and replaced by the newly divided cells.

Stratum Granulosum

In the stratum granulosum, the cells appear in various stages of degeneration and as a rule, break down, and cell death occurs. It is in the stratum granulosum that keratin, a waterproofing protein is produced.

Stratum Lucidum

This is more pronounced in the thick skin of the palms and soles of the feet. This layer consists of 3-4 rows of clear, flat dead cells.

Stratum Spinosum

This layer contains 8-10 closely fitted rows of polyhedral cells. These cells are able to synthesize protein but they cannot reproduce.

Stratum Germinativum

This inner most layer is composed of columnar cells, which are capable of continued cell division. They are anchored to the basement membrane by adhesive molecules, namely fibronectin. These immature cells continuously divide and migrate towards the surface to replace the dead surface cells. The same type of regenerating epidermal cells are found in hair follicles and other skin appendages, which are anchored in the dermis. Other cell types in the mature epidermis are:

A. *Melanocytes* are the pigment producing cells of neuroectodermal origin. These cells synthesize melanin from tyrosine, a pigment responsible for skin color and essential for protection from ultraviolet (UV) light-induced cell damage. It is the amount of malanin in keratinocytes which determines skin color. The absolute number of melanocytes is the same in individuals of greatly differing skin tone. Racial differences in color are the result of metabolically active melanocytes with more dendritic connections.

B. *Langerhan cells* are the macrophage-like antigen-processing cells located above the basal layer of keratinocytes, which interact with helper T cells in assisting with the immune response and may be a possible source of protaglandins; and

C. *Meckel's cells* are the non-pigmented dendrocytes containing cytoplasmic dense core granules which function as touch receptors and also interact with suppressor T cells in assisting with the immune response. Endothelial cells are not found since the epidermis lacks blood vessels. Nutrient delivery and waste transport are by diffusion. There are capillary networks in the papillary dermis which provide this function.

EPIDERMAL RIDGES AND GROOVES

Epidermal ridges (finger/toe prints) develop during the 3rd and 4th fetal month, and are unique to each individual. Their purpose is to increase grip by increasing friction by acting like suction cups. The ducts of sweat glands open in these ridges and are responsible for leaving finger/toe prints.

Epidermal grooves divide the surface of the epidermis into diamond-shaped areas, with hairs typically emerging at the points of groove intersection. Epidermal grooves increase in frequency and depth at the joint areas of fingers and toes.

HAIR AND NAILS

Hair and nails are specialized forms of keratinized epidermis. Both are the result of tightly fused epidermal cells undergoing differentiation. The synthesis of both depend on adequate nutrition and are under influence of various hormones.

There are two main types of hair: terminal and villus. Terminal is long, coarse, and visible; villus is almost un-noticeable. Hair growth takes place in cycles, anagen (hair growth) followed by telogen (rest). At any time about 10-15 percent of hair follicles are in a resting, telogen period. The actual period of growth and rest varies with the body region. For example, scalp hairs grow for 3-10 years, involute over several weeks, and then rest for 3-4 months.

BASEMENT MEMBRANE

Basement membrane is a semipermeable membrane between epidermis and dermis. It is acellular and has two layers, *lamina lucida* and *lamina densa* (basal lamina). Lamina lucida (laminin) is a high molecular weight glycoprotein that cements epidermal cells to lamina densa. Lamina densa consists of type IV collagen. It is a non-fiber forming "net-like" sctructure providing support and flexibility. Epidermal cells preferentially attach to the anchoring fibrils extending into dermis. Other components of the basement membrane include KF-I, AF-I, AF-2, Entactin and Types V, VII collagen. Basement membrane provides mechanical support for the epidermis and regulates transfer of materials between dermis and epidermis.

DERMIS

The second, inner layer of the skin is the dermis. It is derived from mesoderm and its thickness varies from 2-4 mm. Dermis is vascularized and innervated. It is composed of connective tissue containing collagenous and elastic fibers which provide strength and elasticity to the dermis and is divided into a thin superficial layer known as the *papillary dermis* and deeper layer known as the *reticular dermis.*

Papillary Dermis

Papillary layer has many small, elongated projections called rete pegs, also contain loops of capillaries and these project into the epidermis. The size and arrangement of the dermal papillae form ridges which are the external surface of the epidermis and provide attachment of the epidermis to the dermis and its collagen fibers. The ridge patterns on the fingertips and thumbs are unique in each individual and these make up our fingerprints. In some of the dermal papillae are present, Meissner's corpuscles, the nerve endings sensitive to light touch.

Reticular Dermis

The remaining area of dermis is the reticular layer. It is made up of dense, irregular, collagenous tissue, which allows for strength and flexibility in every direction. The primary cell of this layer is the fibroblast, which produces the key structure of the extracellular matrix proteins namely collagen and elastin, as well as the matrix or ground substance. These cells produce the key adhesive proteins used to attach epidermal cells to the basement membrane and are used for epidermal cell migration and replication. The fibronectin is a key fibroblast derived signal protein for the orchestration of healing the ground substance or matrix. This is made up of polysaccharide-protein complexes known as glycosamino-glycans or the GAG component as well as hyaluronic acid which is a semi-fluid that allows cells and connective tissue orientation, provides nutrient diffusion to the cells and also provides a scaffolding for cell migration. The spaces between the interfacing connective tissue fibers are occupied by adipose tissue, blood vessels, sweat glands, nerves and hair follicles. The reticular layer is attached to the underlying structure by the subcutaneous layer of tissue.

CELLULAR COMPONENT OF DERMIS

Fibroblasts and Myofibroblasts

Fibroblasts are spindle shaped cells with large nuclei. The cytoplasm contains rough endoplasmic reticulum (RER) which forms sisterns. These cells become active during wound healing/inflammation and synthesize extra cellular matrix. Myofibroblast on the other hand contain contractile microfilaments (Actin) similar to smooth muscle cells and contribute to wound contraction and remodeling.

Macrophages

They are phagocytic cells, arising from vascular monocytes and they also play a role in wound healing by stimulating fibroblasts.

Mast Cells

Mast cells are often present in upper dermis near blood vessels and nerves and may function in regulation of blood flow. Intracellular granules of mast cells produce many compounds, especially, histamine, heparin, proteoglycans, proteases and prostaglandins.

Lymphocytes

Mostly mediate immune function.

Blood Supply

Subdermal *plexus* of vessels supply dermal (middermal) and papillary plexus. A-V shunts are present known as *glomus bodies* for temperature regulation. Dermis has a rich supply of lymphatics.

Sensory Receptors

In addition to free nerve endings, the dermis contains the following special receptors:

Meissner's corpuscles	Texture; localization
Krause's end bulbs	Cold sensation
Ruffini terminals	Heat sensation
Pacinian corpuscles	Vibration; deep pressure

ANATOMY OF THE BURN WOUND

Thermal destruction of the skin results in severe local and systemic alterations. The amount of tissue destruction is based on temperature and time of exposure: Anatomical assessment involves both the extent and depth of the burn wound.

Extent of Burn Wound

Estimation of extent of the burn wound is simplified by the Wallace's "Rule of Nines" and is easily remembered (Figure 1.2). Each upper extremity and the head are 9% of the body's

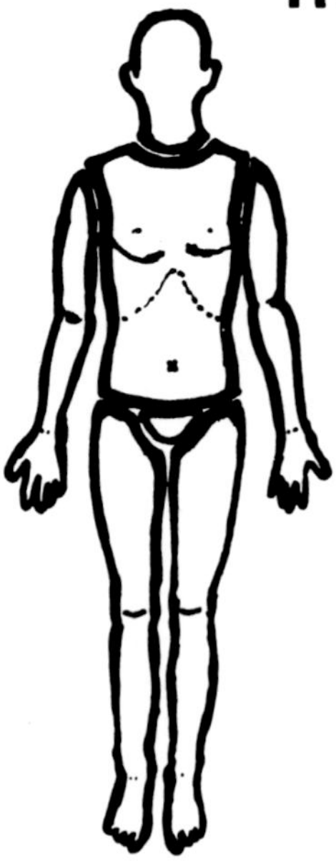

RULE OF "NINES"

Head & Neck	9%
L. Upper Extremity	9%
R. Upper Extremity	9%
Anterior Trunk	18%
Posterior Trunk	18%
L. Lower Extremity	18%
R. Lower Extremity	18%
Perineum	1%

Figure 1.2: Estimation of extent of burn injury: Rule of "NINES"

surface area, each lower extremity, the back and anterior trunk are 18%. The rule of nine is used to estimate the extent of burn injury in adults and is slightly inexact. This method can be used for rapid estimation of extent of burn wounds in adults and in children over 15 years of age. In younger children, the head is proportionately larger, approaching three times the surface area of the adult. Consequently appropriate adjustments must be made in the calculation of burn wound size (**Figure 1.3**). For smaller burns one can estimate the size of the injury using a single surface of the patients hand as 1.25% of the person's body surface area; however, in the larger burns, use of this method may be associated with an error up to 10%. A diagram of the wound with special emphasis on the distribution of the injury is essential. Any adaptation of Lund-Browder chart for recording the extent of burn wound is very useful in both adults and children (**Figure 1.4**).

Depth of Burn Wound

Human skin can tolerate temperatures up to 40°C (104°F) for relatively long periods of time before apparent injury. Temperatures above this level, however, produce a logarithmic increase in tissue destruction. The degree of tissue destruction correlates with both temperature and duration of exposure to the heat source (**Figure 1.5**). Thus the depth of burning is determined by a combination of the burning agent, the temperature, and the time of exposure.

Burns have been described classically into first degree, second degree and third degree injuries, with respect to depth the more descriptive terms being partial thickness and full

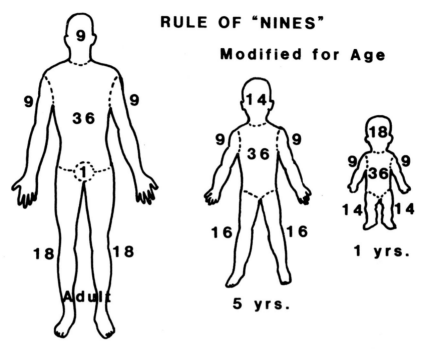

RULE OF "NINES"

Modified for Age

9

9   36   9

1

18   18

Adult

14

9   36   9

16   16

5 yrs.

18

9   36   9

14   14

1 yrs.

Figure 1.3: Estimation of extent of burn injury: Rule of "NINES" modified for age

AREA	INFANT	1-4	5-9	10-14	15	ADULT	PARTIAL	FULL	TOTAL	DONOR AREA
HEAD	19	17	13	11	9	7				
NECK	2	2	2	2	2	2				
A-TRUNK	13	13	13	13	13	13				
P-TRUNK	13	13	13	13	13	13				
R-BUTT	2½	2½	2½	2½	2½	2½				
L-BUTT	2½	2½	2½	2½	2½	2½				
GENITAL	1	1	1	1	1	1				
R-U-ARM	4	4	4	4	4	4				
L-U-ARM	4	4	4	4	4	4				
R-L-ARM	3	3	3	3	3	3				
L-L-ARM	3	3	3	3	3	3				
R-HAND	2½	2½	2½	2½	2½	2½				
L-HAND	2½	2½	2½	2½	2½	2½				
R-THIGH	5½	6½	8	8½	9	9½				
L-THIGH	5½	6½	8	8½	9	9½				
R-LEG	5	5	5½	6	6½	7				
L-LEG	5	5	5½	6	6½	7				
R-FOOT	3½	3½	3½	3½	3½	3½				
L-FOOT	3½	3½	3½	3½	3½	3½				
TOTAL:										

Figure 1.4: Estimation of extent of burn injury: Lund-Browder chart

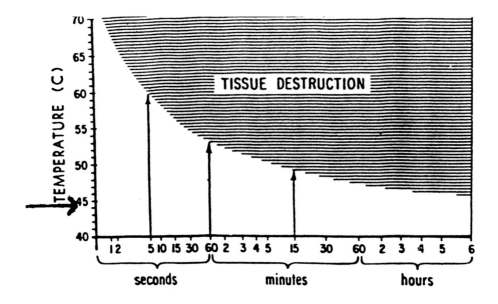

Figure 1.5: Temperature duration curve. Skin destruction proceeds logarithmically with increasing temperatures as a function of time exposure

Table 1.1: Differential diagnosis of depth of burn

	Partial thickness burn	*Full thickness burn*
Sensation	Normal or increased sensitivity to pain and temperature	Anesthetic to pain and temperature
Blisters	Large, thick-walled; will usually increase in size	None or thin-walled; will not increase in size.
Color	Red, will blanch with pressure and refill	White, brown, black, or red; if red, will not blanch with pressure
Texture	Normal or firm	Firm or leathery

thickness burns (**Table 1.1**). Despite modern technology, clinical observation still remains the standard for assessment of depth of the burn wound. Observing the color and texture of the burn as well as the presence of blisters assesses the depth. An assessment of sensation in the wound is also helpful (*see* **Figure 1.1B**).

First Degree Burns

Involves the epidermis only with mild erythematous alteration of the skin with no blister formation such as sun burns in individuals with light colored skin. The desiccated outer layers of epidermis peals of in one to two weeks time and heals with out any residual scar formation (**Figure 1.6**).

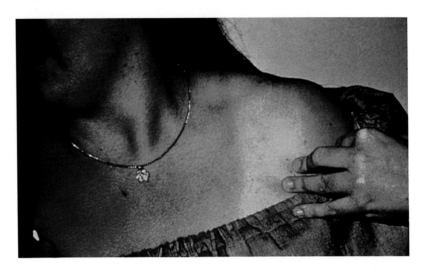

Figure 1.6: First degree burn an example of sun burn with erythema and with no blisters

Second Degree Burns

Partial thickness burns Second degree burns on the other hand involves entire epidermis and part of the dermis that is involved in dermal necrosis. Depending on the depth of injury into the dermis they are divided into two subgroups namely superficial second degree (superficial partial) and deep second degree (deep partial) burns.

Superficial partial burns These burns consist of severe erythematous appearance of the skin with blister formation. Prominent edema causes the wound surface to be elevated above the surrounding unburned skin. Histologically, there may be hygroscopic swelling of the epithelial nuclei and superficial adnexa, and chromatin is displaced toward one side of the nucleus. More severe lesions may lead to actual nuclear pyknosis and cytoplasmic vacuolization. The erythema is due to hyperemia of superficial dermal capillaries with occasional extravasation of erythrocytes. Collagen fibers may be separated by edema. In the absence of any complications these burns will heal spontaneously within three weeks with minimal or no scaring (**Figure 1.7**).

Deep partial burns These burns are characterized by a soft, dry, waxy, white appearance after devitalized material is removed. The tissue is not initially edematous and is not sensitive to pin prick, but perception of deep pressure is still intact. Histologically, necrosis occurs in both the dermis and epidermis. The epithelial nuclei show marked pyknosis and cytoplasmic alteration. Development of inter cellular edema causes detachment of the basal cells from the epidermal basement membrane and leads to formation of a subepidermal bulla. The basal cells soon become detached from surrounding cells and some may be observed with the blister fluid. The dermal injury consists of progressive eosinophilia, swelling and fusion of collagen fibers. Blood vessels especially venules within the dermis, are occluded by thrombi

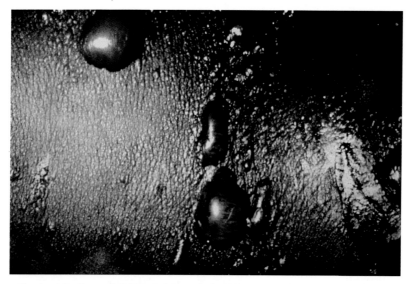

Figure 1.7: Superficial 2nd degree (superficial partial) burns with blisters

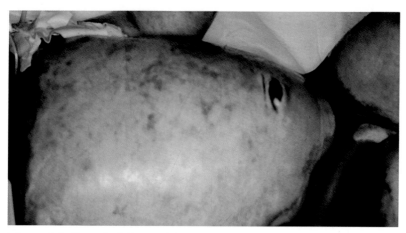

Figure 1.8: Deep 2nd degree (deep partial) burns. Moist with marble white
appearance and edematous

which are predominantly erthrocytic in composition. Deep partial thickness burns may destroy
some of the adnexa structures, but the capacity for spontaneous healing though prolonged is
still present (Figure 1.8).

Third Degree (Full Thickness) Burns

These burns are characterized by a white to black hard, "Leathery" inelastic eschar that may
have a glistening, apparently translucent surface. The wound is insensitive to all but deep
pressure. Coagulative necrosis affects the entire thickness of the epidermis and dermis and

usually extends into subcutaneous fat. These changes result in prominent shrinkage of both the nucleus and cytoplasm of each epithelial, fat and connective tissue cells within the affected area. Deep dermal and subcutaneous blood vessels often contain thrombi. Because of the varying sensitivity of different tissues to injury, collagen which appears viable may be intermixed with necrotic adnexal structures in the early post-burn period. This arrangement complicates differentiation of deep partial thickness burns from full thickness burns. It is possible to have both partial and full-thickness components in the same burn wound. Such wounds are called "Mixed" or burns of indeterminent depth. It is also possible for partial thickness burns to be asensate. When using pain as a factor in determination of depth of injury, however, the response is useful only when it is positive because of neurapraxia of the nerve ending in the skin after the burn injury **(Figure 1.9)**.

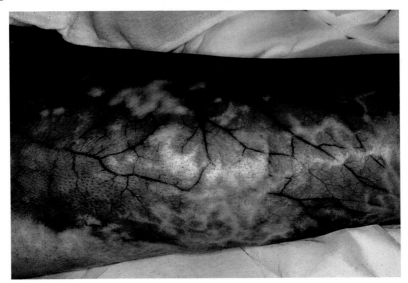

Figure 1.9: 3rd degree (full-thickness) burns with dry eschar and thrombosed dermal and subdermal blood vessels (burn angiogram) a classical sign of full-thickness burn injury

FUNCTIONAL ZONES OF THE BURN WOUND

Close observation of the burn wound demonstrates three separate "Functional Zones" in the immediate post burn period, described by Jackson **(Figure 1.10)**.
1. Zone of coagulation
2. Zone of stasis
3. Zone of hyperemia

Zone of Coagulation

This zone is composed of the surface tissue necrosis with denatured protein and coagulated blood vessels in the initial burn eschar. The surface injury is caused by the heat or the chemical insult. Obviously this zone has an irreversible injury.

THREE ZONES OF THE BURN WOUND

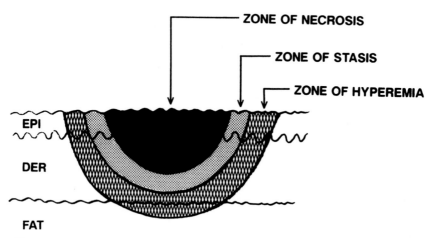

Figure 1.10: Jackson's classic description of three zones of major burn injury

Zone of Stasis

This is an area deep and peripheral to the zone of coagulation where there is impaired circulation. This is a sizable area of tissue injury where cells are viable but can easily be further damaged. Progressive injury in this area was thought to be due to capillary thrombosis from the injured tissue, leading to ischemia induced cell death. This zone is most prominent in deep partial burns where there is less reserve of remaining viable cells and less blood flow.

Zone of Hyperemia

This is an area peripheral to and beyond the zone of stasis. This area is characterized by minimal cell injury, vasodilatation and increased blood flow. This response is probably due to neighbouring inflammation induced mediators. Complete recovery of the tissue healing in this zone is usually expected.

RECENT ADVANCES IN THE ASSESSMENT OF BURN DEPTH

Search for more precise diagnosis of burn depth is going on, since it became important to determine whether the patient with burns of indeterminent depth would benefit from early surgical excision and wound closure. A number of methods have been used based on the physiological changes that occur in the skin after burning and the ability to detect dead cells and denatured collagen.

Wound Biopsy

Histological wound biopsy would seem to be the most precise diagnostic tool, however, biopsies are rarely used in clinical practice. Burn wound is dynamic during the first week of injury and to obtain reproducible results, one has to wait until the end of 1st week. Biopsy results in permanent scars on partial thickness burns. They require experienced pathologist to detect live from denatured collagen and cells. They are expensive. Hence biopsy studies are useful in research studies only and are not applicable for clinical practice.

Ultrasound

Using ultrasonic scanning techniques, some investigators were able to detect denatured collagen in experimental pig model. The problem with this method is that collagen denatures at 65°C, while the epidermal cells, from which burns must heal are killed at about 45°C. As a result the apparent depth is likely to be underestimated by ultrasound. Recent human studies in a small group of patients failed to indicate any improvement in determining the depth of burn compared to the clinical evaluation and histological study of the wound biopsy in the same area.

Vital Dyes

A vital dye directly applied to the burn wound would be useful in detecting dead tissue and also in determining the depth of excision. Ideally the dye should stain only dead tissue, not to be removable with wound care, be nontoxic, provide sharp demarcation between living and dead tissue, penetrate all the dead tissue, and be compatible with topical agents usually used on the burn wounds. Many vital dyes were evaluated in animal models and methylene blue which is metabolized to a colorless compound by living cells was selected with encouraging results in the primary study; however clinical study in a small group of patients did not produce a satisfactorily sharp demarcation to guide excision.

Altered Blood Flow

India Ink

In experimental small animal models India ink can provide one time demonstration of blood flow to the skin. India Ink, however, kills the animal on injection: so, while useful as an experimental technique, it has no role in clinical wound management.

Fluorescein Fluorometry

Fluorescein injected systemically, is delivered through a patent circulation and fluoresces under ultraviolet light. It has been widely used to determine the viability of skin flaps. The use of flourescein fluorescence to determine the burn depth was first reported in 1943. Further refinements in this technique were made recently to measure the magnitude of fluorescence using a fibroptic perfusion fluorometer and high speed Polaroid photography. This technique is best at distinguishing full thickness (no fluorescence) from partial thickness burns where there is little confusion in clinical diagnosis, but it can not distinguish between intermediate and deep dermal burn, where the distinction is crucial in surgical management of the wound.

Laser Doppler Flowmetry

Laser Doppler has been used since 1975 for monitoring cutaneous circulation. Sorensen's group in Denmark first reported the use of a laser Doppler in burn patients. Initial studies showed excellent correlation with full thickness burns (no flow) and partial thickness burns (normal or increases flow). Clinical studies using the laser Doppler to determine burn depth are on going, and refinement of the technology continue; however, its use has not become standard in every day clinical decision making to graft or not to graft.

Thermography

This technique is based on the fact that diminished blood flow to deep dermal and full thickness burns make them cooler to touch, a finding confirmed by thermography. Thermography, like the laser Doppler is highly dependent on room and patient temperature, the patient anxiety and stress level and area of the body considered. Despite these drawbacks clinical studies comparing thermography to clinical assessment proved to be promising.

Light Reflectance

The skin is relatively transparent to short wavelength infrared light and reduced hemoglobin absorbs more of the light than oxygenated hemoglobin. Thrombosed vessels in full thickness burns would become visible in infrared light and could be distinguished from the open vessels of partial thickness burns. Computer analysis of infrared photographs taken with red, green and infrared filtered light may accurately distinguish intermediate, deep dermal and full thickness burns. Unfortunately wound analysis was very expensive and time consuming with this method. It is too slow for clinical decision-making.

Physical Changes

Magnetic resonance imaging (MRI)   Full thickness burns result in slower resumption of water edema than partial thickness burns, since proton MRI parameters correlate with tissue water content. Researchers are working to determine whether Proton MRI could distinguish the depth of the burns; however, its usefulness in clinical application is still some time away. Current status of precise determination of burn depth awaits further refinement of instrumentation and clinical assessment still reflects the standard method for use.

CLASSIFICATION OF BURN SEVERITY

Burns are classified as major, moderate, or minor based on their extent, depth, etiology, and location. Associated injuries and other medical problems are also important (Table 1.2). A major burn has any one of the following characteristics: total of 25% or greater. Total-full thickness extent of 10% or greater, associated smoke inhalation, or electrical cause. Any burns to vital or sensitive areas, such as the face, hands feet or perineum, are also considered major burns. In contrast, moderate burns involve less than 25% but more than 15% of the body surface area, or have full-thickness components of 2-10% of body surface area. Any burn of lesser extent is considered minor. Any burns in poor risk patients (those older than 60 or younger

Table 1.2: Severity classification of burns*

Criteria	Major	Moderate	Minor
Total burn	Over 25% (adult) Over 20% (child)	15-25% (adult) 10-20% (child)	Under 15% (adult) Under 10% (child)
Full thickness	Over 10%	2-10%	Under 2%
Location of burns			
Face	Yes	No	No
Eyes	Yes	No	No
Hands	Yes	No	No
Feet	Yes	No	No
Perineum	Yes	No	No
Age	Over 60 years Under 2 years		
Associated injury	Yes	No	No
Pre-existing disease	Yes	No	No
Electrical burn	Yes	No	No
Smoke inhalation	Yes	No	No

* From American Burn Association: Total care of burn patients, a guide to hospital resources. *Bull. AM. Coll. Surg.* 69 (10: 24-28, 1989).

than 2 years of age, and those with preexisting morbidities) are considered major regardless of their extent, depth, or location. Any patient with a major burn should be cared for at a specialized burn center and should be transferred there as soon as possible.

BIBLIOGRAPHY

1. Carrougher GJ: Burn care and therapy. In Rutan RL: *Physiologic Response to Cutaneous Burn Injury.* Seattle, Mosby, 1998.
2. Cimino VG, Krosner SM, Hanumadass ML: *Occupational Medicine State of the Art Review.* Hanley & Belfus, Inc Philadelphia **10:** 4, 1995.
3. Guyton AC: *Textbook of Medical Physiology,* 8th edn. WB Saunders: Philadelphia, 1991.
4. Hanumadass MD, Ramakrishnan M: *Hand Book of Burns Management.* Jaypee Brothers Medical Publishers Pvt Ltd: New Delhi, 1990.
5. Hanumadass ML, Kagan RJ, Matsuda T: Management of Pediatric burns. Vidyasagar D, Sarkin AP (Eds): *Neonatal and Pediatric Intensive Care.* Littleton, MA. PSG Publishing, 1985.
6. Heimbach D, Hann R, Engrav R: Evaluation of the burn wound, management decisions. Herndon DN (Ed): *Total Burn Care.* WB Saunders: Philadelphia, 1996.
7. Marten JA: Acute management of the burned patient. In Demling RH: *Pathophysiological Changes after Cutaneous Burns and Approach to Initial Resuscitation.* WB Saunders Company: Philadelphia, 1990.
8. Panke TW, McLeod Jr. CG: *Pathology of Thermal Injury: A Practical Approach*: Harcourt Brace Jovanovich Publishers 1985.
9. Reginald LR, Staley MJ: Burn care and rehabilitation, principles and practice. In Falkel JE: *Anatomy and Physiology of the Skin.* FA Davis Company: Philadelphia, 1984.
10. Wachtel TL, Kahn V, Frank HA: *Current Topics in Burn Care.* An Aspen Publication 1983.

2

Physiology of the Burn Wound

PHYSIOLOGIC FUNCTIONS OF THE SKIN

The skin and its many structures perform vital functions that maintain homeostasis within the body. An understanding of the normal functions of the skin is essential to understand the body's responses to the impact of thermal injury. The protective covering of the skin helps maintain fluid and electrolyte balance by preventing the loss of fluid to the environment. Sweat glands excrete salt and water to allow for water evaporation in a controlled fashion. Water loss from the skin averages approximately 300-400 ml daily. Similar amounts of water are lost from the respiratory tract also every day.

Protective Barrier

The skin also serves as a protective barrier to prevent the penetration of bacteria, damaging light and potentially harmful substances in the environment. It pads the internal organs, providing a protection from external trauma.

Regulation of Temperature

The regulation of temperature is another function of the skin. The skin helps to cool the body when the temperature rises by radiating the heat flow in the widened blood vessels and by providing a surface area for the evaporation of sweat. This is done by the chemical mediators, histamine, prostaglandin, and bradykinin, found in the skin. These substances activate the vasodilatation effects on the vascular smooth muscles within the capillaries. When the temperature drops, the blood vessels narrow and the production of sweat decreases.

Sensory Function

The sensory function of the skin is accomplished by a net work of nerve endings and sensory receptors which enable the skin to process environmental stimuli, such as the sensation of heat, cold, pain, pressure, itch, tickle and touch.

Immunologic Function

The macrophages present in the skin provide immunological function by engulfing intruding bacteria. The lymphatic system plays an important role in building immunities and providing defense. Mast cells are responsible for the responses of allergic reactions and inflammation.

Defense from viral infection is provided by the protein, interferon, that is produced by leukocytes, fibroblasts and T cells. Interferon impedes viral replication.

Vitamin D Production

The skin manufactures vitamin D which is essential for the absorption and utilization of calcium from the gastro-intestinal tract.

Identity

Lastly, the skin provides us the identity. It's shape and contours make up our outward appearance.

PHYSIOLOGY OF POST BURN EDEMA

Massive tissue edema after burns is a complex well- recognized entity (Figure 2.1). Edema in non-burn tissue may well be the result of the hypoproteinemia caused by protein loss into the burn tissue.

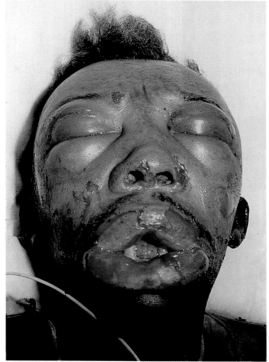

Figure 2.1: Massive edema of the face after burns

Our current knowledge of burn edema formation indicates that the primary process is a severe alteration in the integrity of the microcirculation, resulting in increased loss of fluid and protein into the interstitial space. A second, but apparently less significant, process is an alteration in cell membrane permeability to sodium ion, resulting in a shift of sodium and water into the cells, leading to swelling of the cell. Tissue ischemia due to intravascular fluid loss from the marked increase in microvascular permeability appears to produce the secondary cell membrane alteration.

The degree of increase in transvascular fluid and protein loss after thermal injury is related to both the depth of the burn and the extent of the skin surface involved. The microvascular injury is due, not only to local damage by heat, but also to a number of vasoactive substances released from the burned tissue that act both locally and on the distant microvascular circulation. Edema, therefore, occurs not only in burned tissue, but in nonburned tissue as well. The larger the actual burn area, the more prominent the edema in non-burned tissue. Although the amount of edema in these tissues is significant, the time course and degree of edema formation are considerably less than those found in the area of burn wound itself.

A number of invasive techniques have been used to quantify edema in animal studies including lymph flow and tissue biopsies. However, direct measurement in clinical setting is not possible. Research studies utilizing different techniques have demonstrated that burn edema is maximal usually between 18 and 24 hours. With extensive studies in the past two decades we are beginning to understand the cause of burn wound edema. Ultra structural changes in the microcirculation of thermally injured tissue have been well demonstrated. Even after mild injury, gaps can be seen between endothelial cells as the cells swell and pull apart. Increased protein transport probably occurs, across these gaps. Still, there is a controversy that revolves around the significance of direct vessel injury, versus that produced by vasoactive substances released from the burn. It appears to be well accepted that most mediators effect almost exclusively small vessels, producing gap formation and increasing permeability. There appears to be reasonable evidence that the very early edema formation may be caused by the effect of mediators, particularly histamine, released from the burned tissue into the vessels. This issue as to whether the capillary injury, seen several hours after burn and continuing for even days, is mediators induced or due to direct heat damage remains unresolved.

Another factor postulated by some investigators, to be resolved is about the significance of increased intravascular hydrostatic pressure on the microcirculation of burn tissue. This could result from the arterial dilatation seen in such tissue. When systemic arterial pressure remained constant a relative decrease in arteriolar resistance; riases the hydrostatic pressure. The addition of even a small increase in pressure to a small capillary will increase permeability markedly and that will accentuate the edema process.

BIOCHEMICAL MEDIATORS OF THE BURN WOUND

Many potent vasoactive mediators are known to be released from burn tissue. These include the vasoconstrictors and vasodilators, prostaglandins, kinins, serotonin, histamine, oxygen radicals, and various lipid peroxidases. These factors play a part in postburn inflammation and to some extent edema formation. However, the use of specific systemically administered inhibitors to modify the burn edema process has been unsuccessful. Plasma-exchange transfusions, have occasionally been used in the early post burn period in an attempt to remove these circulating agents. Topically applied inhibitors may be more successful if sufficient concentration of the agents, can be produced in the ischemic burn wound.

Histamine

Histamine is released in large quantities from mast cells in burned skin immediately after injury. This agent has been clearly demonstrated to increase the leakage of fluid and protein permeability from systemic microcirculation. Its major affect being on venules. The increase in histamine levels after burn however, is very transient, indicating that this agent may be involved only in the early increase in permeability. This role is believed by many investigators to be relatively insignificant primarily because of the lack of effect of antihistamines on this process. Only limited success in decreasing edema has been reported with the use of the H_1 receptor inhibitors. Some investigators have reported success in decreasing burn edema using H_2 receptor antagonists in rats pretreated with cimetidine (0.2 mg/gm of body weight). Boykin et al, reported similar findings. Demling observed that pharmacological dose of cimetidine recommended for humans (300 mg, daily) has no effect in reducing edema in burned subjects. It is possible that mega doses of cimetidine are necessary to be effective and the agent must be given immediately after injury.

Prostaglandins

The vasoactive cycloxygenase products of arachidonic acid metabolism, have been reported to be released from burn tissue and, at least in part, to be responsible for the edema formation. Although these substances do not directly alter vascular permeability, it has been suggested that the increased levels of vasodilator prostaglandin, such as PGE_2 and prostacyclin, result in the arteriolar dilatation seen in burned tissue. This would increase the blood flow and intravascular hydrostatic pressure in the injured microcirculation and accentuate the edema process as well. Demling measured levels of the potent vasodilator, PGI_2 and the vasoconstrictor thromboxane, A_2, TXA_2, as their metabolites, in lymph from both burned and non-burned soft tissue and plasma. Levels of PGI_2 were significantly, but not only transiently, increased in non burn lymph with return toward baseline after 12 hours, corresponding with the return of microvascular integrity to normal. Marked and sustained increases in lymph PGI_2 and lymph flow and a severe alteration in permeability were seen in the burned tissue. The injured endothelial cells are most likely source of the increased levels of prostacyclin. Thromboxane was not found to be increased. Inhibition of prostaglandin synthesis has produced variable results. It may well be that several hours after the burn, microcirculation is maximally dilated and is minimally affected by circulating vasodilators. The macrocirculation in the eschar itself is thrombosed, the edema being formed from the injured, vessels in the subeschar region.

Kinins

Kinin, specifically Bradykinin, is known to increase vascular permeability, but primarily in venules. Kinin play a major role in the inflammatory process. Pretreatment with Aprotinin, a protease inhibitor, significantly decreased the free Kinin levels, but appears to have no effect on the edema process. Some researchers have reported a limited decrease in burn edema formation with indirect inhibition of Bradykinin synthesis using a blocking agent.

Serotonin

Serotonin is also released after burns, the exact source is undetermined, but platelets sequestered in the microcirculation are certainly one source. This agent may increase edema by increasing venous resistance and therefore by increasing capillary hydrostatic pressure in the injured vessel. But antiserotonin blockers have been shown non effective in reducing edema as well.

Lypoxygenase Pathway Products

Hydroperoxy fatty acids and the leukotrines are products of this pathway. These products are released after tissue injury and play a major role in the inflammatory response. Leukotrines are potent veno constrictors, and there is some evidence that some of these may also increase permeability.

Free Oxygen Radicals

It has been shown that oxygen free radicals play a key role in increased capillary permeability after burn injuries. It is believed that after major trauma or burn injury a cytokine cascade is activated ,with subsequent stimulation of phagocytic cells for the formation of oxygen free radicals leading to lipid peroxidation. Thomson *et al*, have demonstrated that superoxide dismutase an antioxidant reduces lipid peroxidation, in the immediate post burn period in humans. Vitamin C is another natural antioxidant capable of scavenging superoxide, hydroxyl radicals and singlet oxygen. One of the authors research group have shown that the hourly infusion rate of the resuscitation fluid can be reduced by 75 percent when the Vitamin C (14.2 mg/kg/hr) is administered simultaneously until 24 hours after burn injury and microvascular leakage of fluid and protein can be reduced in the experimental animals.

PHYSIOLOGY OF BURN WOUND HEALING

The burn wound is variable with respect to surface area involved and depth of the injury. Because of their size, partial thickness burn wounds heal by secondary intention. Like all wounds of the skin the primary concern of the burn wound appears to be the effectual restoration of the epidermal barrier which prevents fluid loss and microbial invasion. In order to maintain the regenerated epidermis, the healing process is likewise directed towards the restoration of a supportive dermis with adequate vascular supply and tensile strength to resist wear and tear. By definition full-thickness burns with lack of epithelial source does not heal spontaneously.

The burn wounds do not appear to be much more complicated with respect to healing than other injuries to the integument. Likewise the phases of burn wound repair are similar, if not identical to those observed in other large wounds of the skin.

Inflammatory Phase

All wounds respond to injury with an inflammatory phase. This stage is characterized by initial hemostasis followed by the inflammatory process with migration of polymorphonuclear leukocytes, macrophages and lymphocytes. This phase has the teleological purpose of protecting the tissue from further injury and from microbial invasion. As long as a wound remains open, that is without an epithelial coverage, the wound will remain in this inflammatory process. The longer a wound remains open, the greater will be the degree of inflammation, so too, the longer and more intense the inflammation, the greater will be the degree of scarring. The initial reparative process of phase one will prepare the wound for the connective tissue repair and epithelial cell proliferation (Figure 2.2).

Proliferative Phase (Fibroplasia)

The granulation tissue that is formed after a burn wound consists of a complex tissue which is composed of fibroblasts, capillary networks and other infiltrating cells. The initiation of granulation tissue formation occurs at the time of injury, although the first visible signs of granulation do not appear for two to three days postburn. The first indications are the proliferation of the capillary networks at the base and margins of the wound which results in the bright red coloration of the tissue. Little is known about the factors that stimulate this vascular growth. It has been postulated that reduced blood pressure, and low PO_2 in the wound, changes in the ground substances, metabolic changes and mast cell stimulation are known to be factors that promote the response. The vascular proliferation is accompanied by fibroblasts migrating into the wound tissue and producing new extracellular materials namely collagen, principally with some mucopolysaccharides initially. Likewise macrophages from the blood migrate through the area and remove the debris. Unlike the regimented arrangement of collagen in normal skin, collagen filaments found in burn granulation tissues are characteristically irregularly and angularily shaped.

Restoration of Epidermis

The restoration of epidermis is affected by the mitotic activity of basal cells located in the stratum spinosum of undamaged normal epithelium. The cell division occurs at the wound margin and or from identical areas of skin appendage (hair follicles and sweat glands) remnants located within the wound itself. The zone of mitotic activity seldom exceeds one millimeter width back from the edge of the wound and appears to be unaffected by the size of the wound or severity of injury. The epidermal mitotic activity becomes apparent with in 42 hours after burn with hair follicles appearing to be the most important source of epidermal cells. The mitotic activity of the regenerative epidermis appears to demonstrate a diurnal rhythm with the greatest activity during rest and sleep. This could account for the rarity of mitotic figures that can be observed in burn wound biopsies. After the cell division the new daughter cells appear to detach, flatten considerably and migrate over the wound surface until they cover over the entire wound, if a crust or blister is present, the cells, migrate through the base of the blood and fibrin material of the crust over the reticular layer of the dermis. The production of fibrinolytic or proteolytic enzymes by these cells allow them to

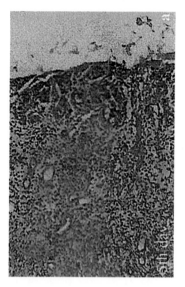

Figure 2.2A: Day 5—Intense localized inflammatory response with neutrophil accumulation

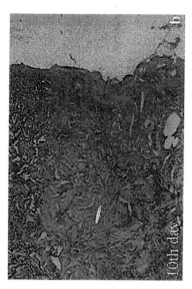

Figure 2.2B: Day 10—Inflammation persisted on this day

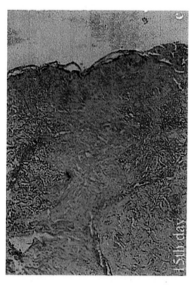

Figure 2.2C: Day 15—Very few capillaries are seen with invasion of inflammatory polymorphic cells and moderate proliferation of fibroblasts

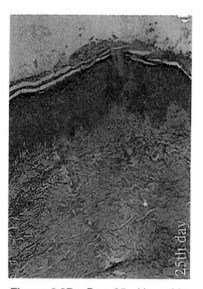

Figure 2.2D: Day 25—Very thin epidermal layer which is not fully differentiated. Less collagen bundles observed in the dermis

Figure 2.2: Histological appearance at various stages of burn wound healing

migrate through the base of the crust material. Within the blister of a second degree burn the rate of epithelization appears to be twice that is seen in similar desiccated areas. The migration of the epidermal cells and their eventual coverage of the wound does not appear to depend upon the presence of a basement membrane which is later formed by the epidermis irrespective of dermal activity. The differentiation of the migrated epidermal cells then reforms the scar epidermis.

As new epidermal cells can only migrate an estimated one centimeter from the site of cell division then, the large full thickness burn that lacks skin appendages must be provided with sources of epidermal cells. This is usually accomplished by grafting procedures.

Repair of the Dermis

The repair of dermis is mediated primarily by the very numerous fibroblasts observed in wound healing tissue. Fibroblasts synthesize the collagen, glycoproteins and mucopolysacharides, that comprise the dermal fibers which provide tensile strength to the integument. The origin of the fibroblast remains some what speculative, but it appears that they do not originate from large monocytes and or macrophages which enter the wound from the blood. It is more probable that they are derived from resting fibrocytes that are found in the adjacent loose subcutaneous tissue, the adventitia of small blood vessels or cells in the fatty tissue.

Maturation Phase

During maturation or remodelling phase of healing, the collagen fibers line up and wave themselves into a fabric of strength. They tend to line up parallel to the "lines of stress" such as across a joint. This process may last for several months to years. This collagen matrix also tend to shorten, such that deformation can be anticipated.

Wound Contraction and Scar Contracture

When the margins of the wound move inwards to effect closure, the process is known as wound contraction. However, burn wounds are usually too extensive to be closed by this activity even though the phenomenon does occur to some extent. Many possible explanations have been proposed for this movement, with two being the most plausible. The first suggests that active cells within the margin of the wound migrate inward pulling on the material within the margins of the defect. This is known as the "Picture Frame Theory"'. However, another explanation might be the "Pull Theory" in which material (collagen fibers and the cells) within the defect, pull on the wound margins. Many workers favor the later concept. We know now that the myofibroblasts present at the base of the wound plays a significant role in the contraction of the wound. Any adjacent skin that is stretched by wound contraction is thinned but is later restored to full thickness by a process known as "Intussusceptive Growth".

Scar

Burn wound contraction often continues with respect to time, beyond the actual closure of the wound. This closure may either be affected by normal repair and/or split-thickness skin grafting. When this happens the scar becomes thick and may result in a disfiguring "Scar Contracture", especially in joints that underlie the tissue. Thus scar contractures are in actuality unabated wound contractions. The contractile myofibroblasts appear to be responsible for both wound contraction and scar contracture.

GROWTH FACTORS IN WOUND HEALING

Cells communicate to each other through the use of specific molecules which are usually proteins. The proteins that are used for cellular communication are called "cytokines". Cytokines are secreted in minute quantities from one cell and then attach to a cellular receptor on another cell (or themselves) to cause a change in the recipient cell. When a protein is released into the blood stream, it acts at an area away from the original cell in what is called an "endocrine" response. When a cell secretes a protein to stimulate a nearby cell, the response is called a "paracrine" interaction. Proteins can be released from a cell which bind to its own receptors in an "autocrine" response. Finally, certain cytokines remain attached to the cell membrane and the interaction involves one cell to another through direct cell contact (juxtacrine" interaction). "Growth factors" are cytokines that specifically stimulate the proliferation of cells. Growth factors can improve wound healing through several mechanisms. First of all, growth factors attract inflammatory cells and fibroblasts into the wound through a process called "chemotaxis". Second, growth factors act as mitogens to stimulate cellular proliferation. Third, growth factors can stimulate the ingrowth of new blood vessels, a process called "angiogenesis". Fourth, growth factors have a profound effect on the production and degradation of the extracellular matrix. Finally, growth factors influence other cell's production of cytokines and growth factors.

There are currently scores of growth factors that have been discovered. A brief summary of some of the more common growth factors will be reviewed. The names of growth factors are frequently misleading because they were often names based on the original cell that they were found to stimulate, the original cell they were produced from, or with what specific assay they were identified. Frequently the names have very little relationship to the actual function of the growth factor.

Platelet-derived Growth Factor (PDGF)

One of the earliest growth factors discovered was PDGF, a growth factor that is a product of not only platelets but macrophages and many other cell types. PDGF exists as a dimer consisting of either an A or a B chain. The most common form in the human platelet is the AB form. PDGF is chemotactic for fibroblasts, smooth muscle cells, and possibly monocytes, and neutrophils. PDGF is a mitogen for smooth muscle cells and fibroblasts. It also has profound effects on the extracellular matrix.

Fibroblast Growth Factor (FGF)

Currently there are at least nine members of the fibroblast growth factor family. These growth factors all have heparin binding capabilities. The first two discovered were acidic and basic FGF and the majority of the healing studies involved these two growth factors. Acidic and basic FGF have profound angiogenic activities. One of the more recently discovered heparin-binding growth factor, keratinocyte growth factor, has been found to have profound stimulatory effect on keratinocyte growth.

Transforming Growth Factor β (TGF- β)

One of the most important growth factor has been the Transforming Growth Factor-β family, which currently consists of five types. Only three are found in the human. The best characterized is TGF-β1, which has been found to have varying effects, depending on the cell type and the environment. TGF-β1 is a very potent stimulant for collagen deposition and inhibits collagen breakdown. Studies do show that if TGF-β1 is blocked, the scar production may be decreased. Interestingly, TGF-β3 may actually inhibit scar formation on its own. TGF-β1 is also very important for the regulation of inflammation. Animals deficient in TGF-β1 expire from an overwhelming inflammatory response. TGF-β is also important for down regulating the growth of many cell types and has been found to be involved in cancer formation when it is not regulated properly.

Epidermal Growth Factor

Epidermal growth factor is a stimulant of all types of epithelial cells. It is a stimulant of epithelial migration and proliferation, and topical application improves healing of partial thickness skin wounds.

Insulin-like Growth Factors (IGF-I, IGF-II)

The Insulin-like growth factors are similar in structure to pro-insulin. They also can bind to the insulin receptor. IGF-I has profound effects on stimulating growth, especially the secondary growth characteristics of adolescence. It also is very important in promoting protein synthesis. The current studies using growth hormone suggest that the anabolic mechanisms of growth hormone act through increases in serum levels of IGF-I. IGF-I also increases the proliferation of many cell types, including fibroblasts; however, it frequently needs to be combined with another growth factor such as PDGF or FGF. IGF-II is felt to be more active in fetal growth; however, it has been found to have similar effects as IGF-I and also can improve healing.

Studies Supporting the Role of Growth Factors in Wound Healing

Growth factors have been found to improve healing in almost all kinds of wounds. Most healing occurs without problems unless there is some form of host impairment such as diabetes, malnutrition, infection, or after treatment with steroids, chemotherapy agents, or radiation. Several studies have demonstrated that growth factors can improve healing in animals impaired with diabetes, malnutrition, infection, or after treatment with chemotherapy agents, steroids, and radiation. Since multiple growth factors are present in the wound, some studies have focused on determining whether growth factor combinations can enhance healing to a greater extent than a single growth factor. The rationale behind doing such studies is that *in vitro* studies suggest that more than one growth factor may be required for a cell to enter the cell cycle.

The Role of Growth Factors in Burn Wound Healing

It is important to remember that growth factors may not always be necessary for the normal healing of the burn patient. Growth factors that improve healing of an open wound or an incision may not be appropriate for a burn patient. Most burn patients with deep burns undergo excision and grafting so that studies that examine the role of topical growth factors in contracting a wound are not appropriate for burn patients. Circumstances in which growth factors may have a role in burn patients include the following:
1. Acceleration of donor site healing
2. Healing of partial thickness wounds
3. Healing of hard-to-heal areas such as over exposed tendon or bone
4. Improving the take of skin grafts
5. Improving the take of skin substitutes.

Clinical Studies

Clinical studies have focused on two types of wounds:
1. Healing of chronic nonhealing dermal ulcers - Studies have suggested that several growth factors including PDGF, FGF, EGF, and TGF-β, may improve healing in these chronic wounds.
2. Healing of split-thickness donor sites.

Brown *et al* published the first study suggesting that EGF had the potential to improve healing of burn wound donor sites. They found that the topical application of EGF produced a modest improvement in the time required for healing of these split-thickness donor sites. In essence, it required one to two or fewer days to heal. This study was repeated in normal volunteers by Cohen who found no difference in the rate of epithelial closure. Greenhalgh *et al*, examined the role of basic FGF in improving donor site healing in burned children and found no difference in the rate of closure. Barbul also suggested that there may be a modest improvement in healing in donor sites treated with topical interleukin-I. All these studies suggested that although there was possible improvement in some of the studies, the amount of improvement was not clinically significant. The one study that did show a potentially valuable improvement was in Herndon's systemic growth hormone study. Where the previous studies examined patients with a relatively minor burn, Herndon's group examined patients with burn wounds large enough to require multiple donor site reharvests. With a greater wound burden, healing is probably impaired to the point that growth factors can make a more clinically significant improvement. Herndon found that patients treated with growth hormone had significant shortening of their hospital stay because they are able to reharvest the donor sites days earlier over several grafting procedures. These points are very important since the use of topical growth factors in patients with small burns and small donor sites probably is not of clinical relevance since most of these patients can heal their donor sites quite quickly and frequently can be treated as outpatients. Those patients who may benefit from topical growth factors will be those who have extensive burns and thus who require multiple reharvesting of their donor sites. Shortening the time for donor site reharvest by even a few days would add up to a significantly shortened hospital stay when multiple grafting procedures are required. The role of growth factors in the other areas have not been extensively examined. Currently, skin substitute take is only fair at best. Growth factors that could improve the take and vascularity of skin substitutes to allow the survival of the keratinocytes would most likely be of benefit. Studies need to continue in these other areas of burn wound healing.

BIBLIOGRAPHY

1. Burns: *Selected Readings in General Surgery* **21**: 4,1994.
2. Cohen S: The epidermal growth factor (EGF). *Cancer* **51**:1789-91, 1983.
3. Davis JH, Sheldon, GF: *Surgery: A Problem Solving Approach*, 2nd edn. Mosby, St. Louis, 1995.
4. Gabbiani G, Hirschell BJ, Ryan GB, *et al:* Granulation tissue as a contractile organ. A study of structure and function. *J Exper Med* **135**:719-34,1972.
5. Greenhalgh DG, Rieman M: Effects of basic fibroblast growth factor on the healing of partial-thickness donor sites. A prospective, randomized, double-blinded trial. *Wound Rep Reg* **2**:113-21, 1994.
6. Greenhalgh DG, Sprugel KH, Murray MJ, Ross R: PDGF and FGF stimulate healing in the genetically diabetic mouse. *Am J Pathol* **136**:1235-46, 1990.
7. Guyton AC: *Textbook of Medical Physiology*, 8th edn, Philadelphia, WB Saunders 1991.
8. Heldin CH, Ostman A, Westermark B: Structure of platelet-derived growth factor: Implications for functional properties. *Growth Factors* **8**:245-52, 1993.
9. Herndon DN, Barrow RE, Kunkel KR, *et al:* Effects of human growth hormone on donor-site healing in severely burned children. *Ann Surg* **212**:424-31,1990.
10. Hunt TK, Twomey P, Zederfeldt B, *et al:* Respiratory gas tensions and pH in healing wounds. Am J Surg **114**:302-07, 1967.
11. Majno G, Gabbiani G, Hirschel BJ, *et al:* Contraction of granulation tissue *in vitro*: similarity to smooth muscle. *Science* **173**:548-50, 1971.
12. Marten JA: Acute management of the burned patient. In Demling RH: *Pathophysiological Changes after Cutaneous Burns and Approach to Initial Resuscitation*. Philadelphia, WB Saunders Company, 1990.
13. Matsuda TH, Shimazaki S, Matsuda H, Abcarian H, Reyes H, Hanumadass M: High dose vitamin C therapy for extensive deep dermal burns. *Burns* **18**:2,1992.
14. McMinn RMH: *Wound healing*. In The Cell in Medical Science. New York, Academic Press, Vol. 4, 1976.
15. Montandon D, Gabbiani G, Ryan GB, *et al:* The contractile fibroblast. Its relevance in plastic surgery. *Plast Reconstr Surg* **52**:286-92, 1973.
16. Peacock E, Van Winkle W: *Surgery and Biology of Wound Repair*. Philadelphia, WB Saunders Co., 1970.
17. Robson MC, Phillips LG, Thomason A, Robson LE, Pierce GF: Platelet-derived growth factor BB for the treatment of chronic pressure ulcers. *Lancet* **339**:23-25,1992.
18. Rotwein P: Structure, evolution, expression and regulation of insulin-like growth factors I and II. *Growth Factors* **5**:3-18,1991.
19. Schultz GS, Jurkiewicz MJ, Lynch JB: Enhancement of wound healing by tropical treatment with epidermal growth factor. *N Eng J Med* **321**:76-79, 1989.
20. Sporn MB, Roberts AB: Peptide growth factors and inflammation, tissue repair, and cancer. *Clin Invest* **78**:329-32, 1986.
21. Van Winkle W: The epithelium in wound healing. *Surg Gynec Obstet* **127**:1089-15, 1968.
22. Van Winkle W: The fibroblast in wound healing. *Surg Gynec Obstet* **124**:369-86, 1967.
23. Van Winkle W: Wound contraction. *Surg Gynec Obstet* **125**:131-42, 1967.
24. Williams WG, Phillips LG: Pathophysiology of the Burn Wound. In Herndon, DN (Eds): *Total Burn Care*, Philadelphia, WB Saunders, 1996.

3

Pathology of the Burn Wound

Burn injury occurs as a result of an energy transfer from a heat source to the body. This can occur by direct conduction or by electromagnetic radiation. Thermal conduction from one object to another occurs along the gradient from higher to the lower temperatures, with the transfer of heat to the later. Many factors greatly alter the response of the human body as a whole to the energy transfers. Conductivity of the local tissue has a major effect upon the rate of loss or gain of thermal energy. For instance, the nerves and blood vessels conduct heat with the greatest ease, where as bone is the most resistant. Other tissues are intermediate. The peripheral circulation will also be a major factor in determining the rate of absorption or dissipation of heat throughout the body. Skin pigmentation and presence or absence of clothing of different pigment densities, the presence or absence of other insulating materials such as hair, natural skin oils and cornified layer of surface epithelium, and total water content of the tissues will be other factors of major importance.

In addition to direct application of heat to the body surface, radiant energy can produce major thermal injury. Such an injury occurs primarily from electromagnetic spectrum, which includes a wide variety of radiant energy forms to which individuals are exposed. Individuals exposed to heat energy source sustain thermal injury characterized by cell death and coagulation necrosis of the tissue. The temperature and duration of exposure and its relationship to the depth of injury has been discussed in the previous chapters.

The vascular destructive nature of the burn wound is evident with the presence of intravascular red cell destruction. Immediately after burning there is a cessation of blood flow through both the arterial and venous channels. This cessation is caused primarily by thrombosis, and in the full thickness burns persists for three to four weeks, at which time it is replaced by neovasculature or granulation tissue. In partial thickness wounds another sequence follows the initial occlusion. In the more superficial wound there is rapid restoration of arterial and venous circulation with in 24 to 48 hours. If the drying of the wound or infection be allowed to occur, circulation is not re-established and extensive thrombosis of the initial wound and marginal wound takes place. This phenomenon is more prominent on the venous side and thus the partial thickness wounds are converted into full thickness injury.

Immediately after burn injury there is a marked increase in capillary permeability which follows a biphasic pattern. The initial phase lasts for approximately 20 minutes and is closely followed by a second phase of much greater magnitude, which last for two to three weeks. However, the major changes in capillary permeability are over within 24 to 30 hours post-burn and the major segment of this with in the first 12 hours, resulting in extensive tissue edema. The pathophysiology of post burn edema formation has been discussed in detail in the previous chapter. The natural course of the burn wound depends upon the depth of the burn injury. The normal stages of uncomplicated partial thickness and full thickness burn wound is summarized in the Table 3.1.

Table 3.1: Natural course of the burn wound

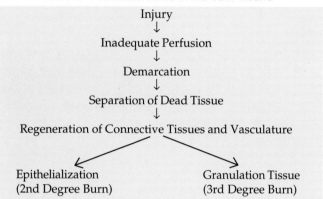

As the acute non-specific inflammatory response reaches its peak two or three days following thermal injury, the small, still functioning vessels regain their integrity and reabsorb the extravasated fluid. Macrophages appear in the area and the invading colonized bacteria secrete collagenase and other proteases, starting the separation of dead tissue from live wound bed (Figure 3.1). The more colonized or infected the wound, the quicker eschar separation occurs. In deeper burns, wound macrophages play a major role in wound healing by releasing multiple factors. Angiogenesis factor is secreted by hypoxic macrophages

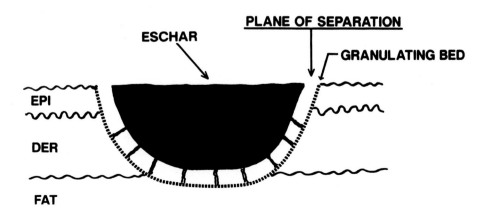

Figure 3.1: Natural separation of eschar in an uncomplicated burn wound

marginated at the wound edges, start neovascularization and granulation tissue formation. Deeper macrophages, with adequate oxygenation, secrete growth factors which stimulate fibroblast proliferation, deposition of collagen, fibronectin and glycosaminoglycan. Excessive bacterial proliferation retards healing through release of excessive proteases. If the wound has not healed with in 14 days, myofibroblasts-fibroblast bundles form and deposits excessive collagen while mast cells release mucopolysaccharides and histamine creating the basis for hypetrophic scar formation.

BURN WOUND INFECTIONS

Infection is a very undesirable event during the management of the burn wound. All burn wounds should be suspected as having wound colonization, until and otherwise proved to the contrary with appropriate culture studies. The gold standard is to eliminate any type of infection, including opportunistic infection during the evolution of wound healing. Burn wound infection can be classified as colonization, non-invasive local infection, invasive wound sepsis and systemic septicaemia.

Colonization

This is defined as a condition where bacterial flora are present on the surface of the burn eschar. They merely show their presence, but do not cause any harm to the patient, though by themselves are pathogenic. Alexander (1987) classified burn wound infection as non-invasive and invasive.

Non-invasive Wound Infection

Local burn wound infection   The infection is limited to burn eschar. It may lead to early separation of eschar and increased purulent discharge from the wound. Infection enters the eschar from the surface through hair follicles.

Invasive Sepsis

Invasive sepsis is defined as the presence of organisms exceeding 100,000 per gram of tissue of the burn area and actively invading the subjacent unburned tissue (Figure 3.2). The sequential progression of bacterial involvement from the surface of the wound to deep unburned tissues has been described by Teplitz (1979).
A. *Supraeschar colonization*   The bacteria are present over the surface of the eschar.
B. *Intrafollicular colonization*   Colonization occurs in the pits of the hair follicles, which are destroyed.
C. *Intraeschar and subeschar colonization*   The micro-organisms invades the coagulated and non-viable tissue.
D. *Invasion of subjacent unburned tissue*   This stage is termed burn wound sepsis. The bacteria colonize along the dermal subcutaneous interface. Perivascular growth leads to thrombosis of vessels and converts deep partial thickness burns to full thickness burns.

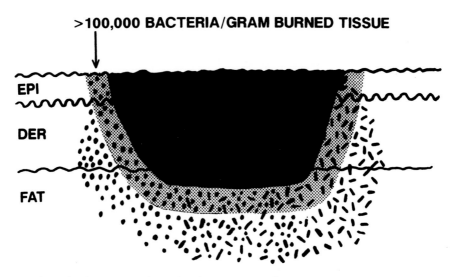

>100,000 BACTERIA/GRAM BURNED TISSUE

EPI

DER

FAT

Figure 3.2: Invasive burn wound sepsis with presence of bacteria in unburned subdermal tissue

Systemic Septicaemia

Here the patient, who suffers from clinical burn wound sepsis, starts manifesting signs of invasion of the blood with offending bacteria. This is a presentation of uncontrolled infection, and toxicity of the bacteria starts manifesting on the various systems of the body. Each bacteria that invades has a definite pattern of toxicity and manifestation, and systemic septicemia may manifest as sudden rise or fall in temperature with chills, rigors, leukocytosis or leukopenia and tachycardia.

Pathological manifestations in sepsis may be the result of both blood stream invasion of organisms and systemic release of exotoxin and endotoxins. Later manifestations of septicaemia are confusion, nausea, vomiting, ileus, hypotension, oliguria and death.

FACTORS PREDISPOSING THE BURN WOUND TO INFECTION

Many factors predispose the burn wound to infective complications and influence the outcome. They are: (a) Injury related, (b) Patient related, (c) Bacteria related and (d) Systemic response related factors.

Injury Related Factors

The extent of injury and depth of burn has a definite bearing on the incidence of infection in burn wounds. Avascularity of full-thickness burn with associated systemic shock and the presence of protein rich eschar promote bacterial proliferation and occurrence of sepsis.

Patient Related Factors

Extremes of age, preexisting chronic disease like diabetes mellitus, immunologic deficits and patients on cytotoxic agents are more prone to infective complications after burn injury.

Bacterial Factors

Microbial factors influencing the increase in the incidence of infections of the burn wounds include, microbial density and composition of the colonizing bacterial flora. The virulence of the bacteria in the wound and release of endotoxin or exotoxin from these bacteria causes systemic sepsis and illness.

Systemic Responses

Major burn injury results in alteration of hormonal milieu of the host, with increase in catecholamines, corticosteroids, glucagon, and decrease in circulating levels of insulin, growth hormone and melatonin. These hormonal changes decrease the host's capacity to fight infections. Release of interleukin -I and tumor necrosis factor will have similar effects in the increase on host's suseptability to sepsis. Certain immunological changes that occur after major burn injury also increases the incidence of sepsis and its outcome. They are: (a) activation of complement via alternative pathway, (b) Depression of circulating levels of immuno-globulins (c) Altered number and function of neutophils and (d) Alteration of lymphocyte populations.

BURN WOUND MICROBIOLOGY

Identification of the pathogens includes the mode of specimen collection, transport media and culture studies. The common specimens taken are the exudates, aspirates, and surface swabs from the burn wound. Tissue biopsy if feasible is the true indicator of identifying the pathogen. If a bacterial count over 100,000 number of microorganisms per gram of tissue is identified, then this is supposed to indicate positive infection. But it is not often necessary to do a quantitative bacterial count, as surface swabs will indicate the organisms when the wound is grossly infected. If microscopic examination of biopsy provides evidence of bacteria in the adjacent unburned tissue, it confirms invasive burn wound sepsis.

Staphylococcus

From the prevalence of the pathogens encountered in Indian Burn Centers, gram-positive *Staphylococcus* tops the list. There are many strains of staphylococci and they have variable hemolytic profile. *Staphylococcus* is the most commonly grown organism.

Coagulase test is a differential test for separating the two types of staphylococci—the *aureus* and the *epidermidis*. Toxic metabolites are produced by both the varieties. Their capacity to developing resistance is also very high. Methicillin resistant staphylococci are also occasionally encountered in the burn centers, but many centers do not give methicillin as an antibiotic in India today.

Methicillin It is semisynthetic penicillin, which is resistant to penicillinase. *Staph. aureus* develops resistance to methicillin very soon, because it produces penicillinase. Methicillin resistance is genetically mediated through a transposon. *Staphylococcus epidermidis* is a resident of human skin and mucous membrane and resembles *Staph. aureus* microscopically. This is also equally pathogenic like *Staph. aureus*. *Staph. epidermidis* also is resistant to penicillinase resistant penicillins. This *Staph. epidermidis* delivers its genetically resistant code to a previously resistant *Staph. aureus*, which subsequently becomes resistant to methicillin. This is then known as MRSA (Methicillin Resistant Staphylococci). This MRSA can be a serious problem, in burn units where the predominant infecting bacteria being *Staph. aureus*. In some burn centers a prophylactic program of methicillin is given (100-gm/kg/body wt given intravenously dissolved in 250 mg. of fluid daily for 21 days after burn). This is supposed to prevent MRSA infection developing. Since methicillin can be given only intravenously, when oral antibiotics have to be continued, oxacillin or nafcillin can be used. In the Indian subcontinent, MRSA is not a problem, because very few centers are using methicillin.

Staphylococcal Septicaemia

The burn wound that has been infected with *Staphylococcus aureus* suddenly appears very exudative and wet **(Figure 3.3)**. There may be purulent discharge. Patient begins to run a high temperature and have leukocytosis. The condition if untreated may result in the patient going into shock with high pulse rate and falling blood pressure. In long standing cases, multiple metastatic abscesses manifest over the skin **(Figure 3.4)**, lung and brain, which may end fatally. The control of fulminating infection is by administering adequate antibiotics after culturing the organism and assessing the sensitivity. As the toxaemia produces severe anemia, repeated small blood transfusions are also beneficial. After the systemic infection gets abated and after surface cultures become negative for the organism, skin grafting, can be undertaken to cover the burn wounds.

Streptococci

These are found less often in the burn wound, and are usually coagulase negative, but produce haemolytic activity in the presence of blood. Clinical features include, exuberant moist granulation tissue

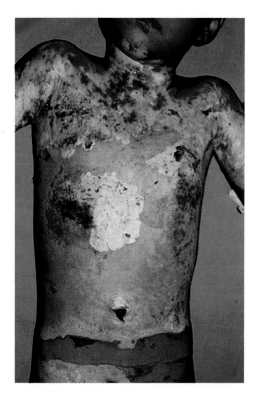

Figure 3.3: Staphylococcal sepsis of the burn wound

with thin serosanguineous discharge **(Figure 3.5)**. Presence of beta-hemolytic streptococci in the wound is associated with repeated graft failures. General condition shows a toxic appearance with leukoctytosis, anemia and high-rise of temperature. This infection coexists with staphylococcal infection. But identification of the pathogen as streptococci is very essential before initiating treatment. Chronic granulating wounds which looks healthy should always be cultured to exclude beta-hemolytic streptococci colonization before skin grafting.

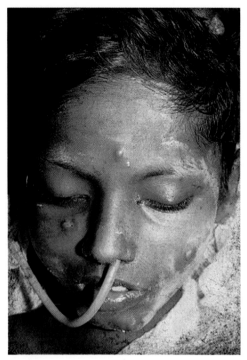

Figure 3.4: Staphylococcal septicaemia with pyogenic abscesses on the face

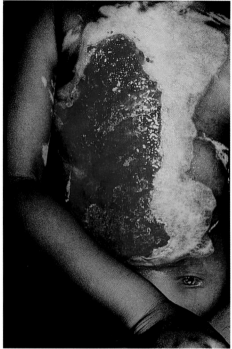

Figure 3.5: Beta-hemolytic streptococcal infection with exuberant red granulation tissue. And scanty discharge. It gives a false appearance of a healthy wound

ANAEROBIC INFECTION

One of the authors reported the occurrence of anaerobic infection in burns, where early closure of the wound has not been done. The anaerobic gram-positive cocci are part of the skin, gastrointestinal tract, genital and oral cavities. The two varieties that are pathogenic are the peptococci and peptostreptococci. These infections are problematic, and the patients appear very ill with high-rise of temperature, and have a peculiar foul smelling discharge, profuse anaemia and an ulcerative wet appearance (Figure 3.6). Special cultures to identify anaerobic bacteria are necessary in the laboratory. The culture swabs are transported in Robertson's cooked meat medium and inoculated into neomycin blood agar first and later into the sugar enriched medium.

Sometimes, clostridium septicum and bacteroids are also grown in these cultures.

CLOSTRIDIAL INFECTION

In electrical burn injuries, where there is avascular muscle tissue, there are chances of clostridial infection. The high risk of developing tetanus even with small burns, have made us give tetanus prophylaxis in the treatment protocol. If prior immunization is unclear, or when the

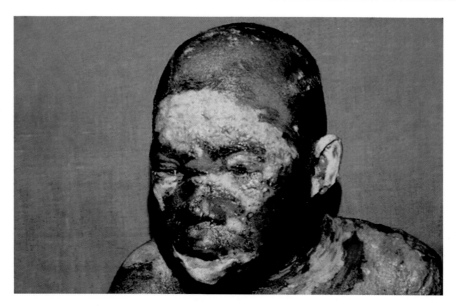

Figure 3.6: Anaerobic bacterial infection of the face and perioral region

patient's booster was more than 10 years ago, 250 units of tetanus anti-serum is given. More important is to remove all the devitalized tissue, and lavage with copious hydrogen peroxide solution and give appropriate antibiotics preferably 4th generation cephalosporins. Currently, prompt and aggressive debridement of non viable tissue in the burn wound and timely performance of escharotomy or fasciotomy have practically eliminated "Gas Gangrene" a rare but dangerous infection caused by *Clostridium* species. These are anaerobic, gram positive, and spore forming bacteria.

ANAEROBIC GRAM-NEGATIVE RODS

The gram-negative bacilli, which are facultative anaerobic rods encountered repeatedly in the burn wound are the *Klebsiella* of the enterobacter group. *Proteus* also is an organism commonly isolated from the burn wound.

ANAEROBIC GRAM-NEGATIVE BACILLI

The most repeatedly confronted organism is the bacteriods species. This can cause very virulent infection. These are found mostly in regions of the orophraynx. This also can cause a picture of anaerobic infection described earlier with anaerobic gram-negative cocci—the peptococci and peptostreptococci.

GRAM NEGATIVE AEROBIC RODS

To this group belongs the *Pseudomonas* species. In the Indian burn centers, burn wound infection with *Pseudomonas aeruginosa* is most common after the staphylococcal infection.

Infection can be of an acute nature and also can lurk as a chronic infection. These organisms use carbohydrates. Where other organisms ferment the carbohydrates, these utilize carbohydrates by oxidation. Though *Pseudomonas* species have been involved in nosocomial infection, the aeruginosa has been recognized as the pathogen in burns. It is also capable of developing resistance rapidly. These organisms usually reside in a burn unit, and enter through contact with fomites. Burn unit staff and care givers often carry the organism and cross contaminate from one patient to the other. The IV portals are a potential source of infection **(Figure 3.7)**. *Pseudomonas* infection can lead on to septicemia. This is a grave condition. Black areas of local discolouration ensue **(Figure 3.8)**. Partial thickness wounds become necrotic and full thickness with greenish blue discharge because of the pigment *pyocinine* it produces **(Figure 3.9)**. The green pus usually associated with burn wound infections by *P. aeruginosa* may represent a favorable sign, suggesting colonization of the eshar or focal, superficial, well controlled infections instead of invasive sepsis. Purplish discolouration and edema surrounding the margin of the wound is a common feature.

Metastatic cutaneous lesions of *P. aeruginosa* known as "Ecthyma Gangrenosum" may appear in concert with, or shortly after invasive infection of the burn wound. These lesions involve burned and unburned skin including skin graft donor sites. These vesicular lesions which are intraepidermal or subdermal leads to necrosis of the epidermis **(Figure 3.10)**. It is usually associated with poor prognosis. Patient gets into septicaemia, with high-rise of temperature, tachycardia, shock and confusion. Leucocytosis is followed by leukopenia and finally the patient gets into a phase of disseminated intravascular coagulopathy with bleeding from the orifices and the situation may end fatally.

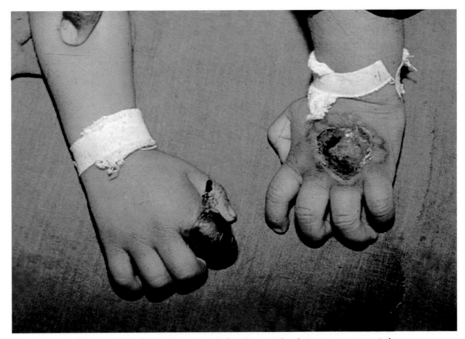

Figure 3.7: *Pseudomonas* infection at the intravenous portal

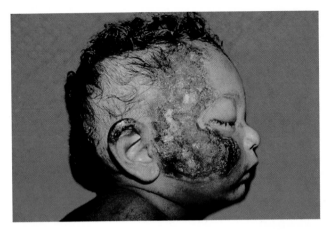

Figure 3.8: *Pseudomonas* infection; bluish-black eschar on a deep partial thickness burn on the face

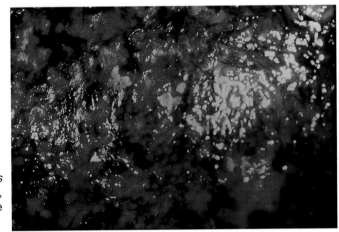

Figure 3.9: Close up view of *Pseudomonas* infected burn wound, showing necrosis, blackish discoloration and greenish-blue discharge

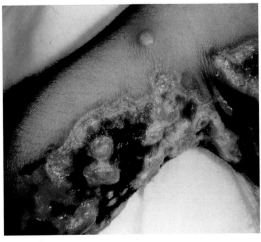

Figure 3.10: *P. Aeruginosa* infection of the burn wound with black necrotic areas. The metastatic cutaneous vesicular lesion over the unburned skin adjacent to the wound is "Ecthyma Gangrenosum" a poor sign of prognosis

FUNGAL INFECTION

In major burn wound infection, one is forced to administer combination antibiotics in an aggressive manner. Under those situations the fungi that are commensals on the skin and in the oral cavity gain access and gets established as burn wound infection. Topical anti-microbial agents also have contributed to the development of super infection with fungi. When the bacteria on the surface of the burn wound become ineffective due to the topical antimicrobials, the lurking inactive fungi becomes active and becomes pathogenic to the burn wound. *Candida* and *Aspergillus* are the two fungi that turns into pathogens. In the case of fungal sepsis, the urine will contain the fungi. But to diagnose an established fungal infection, any one of the three body fluids - urine, blood or wound exudates must culture the fungi. Retinal examination also will reveal the spores. Systemic candidiasis can be fatal. But today fluconazole is very effective in fungal infections. Fungal infection is no more a menace, as it was in the last decade. Repeated graft failures gives an indication of fungal infection, in an otherwise sterile burn wound **(Figure 3.11)**.

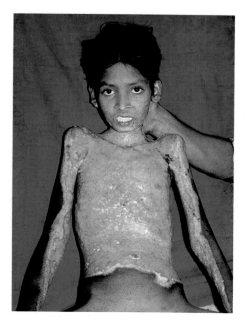

Figure 3.11: *Candida* infection of the burn wound with repeated graft failures

VIRUSES

In extensive burns of over 50 percent TBSA, viral infections are reported. The viruses that infect are the cytomegalovirus (CMV) and the herpes simplex virus. The infection can be fulminating and even may become fatal. One of the sources of infection with virus is due to the multiple blood transfusions that are given for burns, when the virus could have been a contamination. CMV infection typically presents with continued low grade fever and lymphocytosis, in spite of the burn wound having been closed. It can also co-exist with other infections like bacterial and fungal infections. Herpetic infection makes the partial thickness burns converted into full thickness wounds. Distant necrotising lesions may occur in the liver and adrenal glands. Even chicken pox like lesions may manifest in the grafted areas or mucous membrane. If these lesions surface, it is better to wait for re-grafting of the wounds, otherwise graft do not take. Systemic acyclovir can be given for herpetic infections.

Analysis of Burn Wound Infection in KKCTH and Kilpauk Medical College Hospital, Chennai during the year 2000:
A total of 2375 cases were admitted in the hospitals during the year 2000. The policy is to do a surface culture of every burn wounds over 25 percent BSA that is admitted and do a wound biopsy and culture on suspected cases of burn wound infection. 664 cases had a biopsy and quantitative culture done. In this group 427 cases were positive for infection, 388 cases developed invasive sepsis and 338 cases died **(Tables 3.2 to 3.4)**.

Table 3.2

Total number of cases:	2375
Colonization	1711
Biopsy culture	664
Positive biopsy culture	427
Invasive sepsis (100,000 org/gm of tissue)	388
Mortality	338

Table 3.3: Type of infection, depth of burns, and total body surface area- Year 2000

Percentage Total Body Surface Area (%)

Bacteria grown	15-24%		25 - 34%		35 - 45%	
	P.T	F.T	P.T.	F.T	P.T.	F.T.
Staphylococcus auerus	21	50	287	101	112	63
Klebsiella	30	99	103	50	27	20
E. coli	5	30	71	129	31	99
Proteus	9	47	64	44	21	73
Pseudomonas	Nil	Nil	16	57	11	24
Anaerobes	Nil	Nil	Nil	Nil	Nil	18
Fungus	Nil	Nil	Nil	Nil	Nil	Nil

(Local wound infection as well as invasive burn wound sepsis are included in the above study)

Table 3.4: Analysis of wound surface cultures and biopsy cultures

Positive Cultures:			
1. Staphylococcus aureus	634		
2. E. coli	364		
3. Klebsiella	329		
4. Proteus	258		
5. Pseudomonas aeruginosa	108		
6. Anaerobic infections with Peptostreptococci	18		
TOTAL:	1711		
Positive Biopsy Cultures	427	Invasive sepsis	Mortality
1. Staphylococcus aureus	157	148	133
2. E.coli	92	89	76
3. Klebsiella	48	44	36
4. Proteus	73	61	54
5. Pseudomonas aeruginosa	51	43	38
6. Anaerobic infection with Peptostreptococci	6	3	1
Total Number of infected burn wounds	1711		
Total number of biopsy positive wounds	427		
Total number of invasive sepsis	388		
Mortality in invasive sepsis	338		

BIBLIOGRAPHY

1. Alexander JW. The role of infection in the burn patients in *The Art and Science of Burn Care*. Boswick JA (Ed). Anaspen publication, Maryland, USA 103-12; 1987.
2. Banda MJ, Knighton DR, Hunt TK, Werb Z. Isolation of a nonmitogenic angiogenesis factor from wound fluid. *Proc Natl Acad Sci USA* **79:** 7773, 1982.
3. Collentine GE, Waisbren BA, Mellender JW: The treatment of burns with invasive antibiotic therapy and exposure. *JAMA* **200:** 939-42, 1967.
4. Davies DM, Brown JM, Bennett JP *et al*. Survival after major burn complicated by gas gangrene, acute renal failure, and toxic myocarditis. *Br Med J* **1:**718-19,1979.
5. Davies DM. Gas gangrene as a complication of burns. *Scand J Plast Reconstr Surg* **13:**73-75, 1979.
6. Fry DE, Peartstein L, Fultan RL, Polk HC: Multiple system organ failure: The role of uncontrolled infection. *Arch Surg* **115:** 136-140,1980.
7. Hart GB, Lamb RC, Strauss MB. Gas gangrene: I. A collective review. *J Trauma* **23:**991-1000,1983.
8. Herndon DN. Infections in burns. *Total Burn Care* WB Saunders Company Ltd. USA, 98-135.
9. Hunt TK, Andrews WS, Holliday B *et al*. Coagulation and macrophage stimulation of angiogenesis and wound healing. *In: The Surgical Wound* (Driven P, Hildrick-Smith P, Eds). Lea & Febiger, Philadelphia, 1981.
10. Knighton DR, Hunt TK, Scheuenstuhl H, *et al*. Oxygen tension regulates the expression of angiogenesis factor by *Macroph Science* 1983; 1283.
11. Monafo WW, Freedman B. Topical therapy for burns. *Surg Clin N America* **67:**133-45; 1987.
12. Ponder E. The coefficient of thermal conductivity of blood and various tissues. *J Gen Physiol* **45:**545, 1962
13. Pruitt BA Jr, Foley F. The use of biopsies in burn patient care. *Surgery* **73:** 887-97; 1973.
14. Pruitt BA Jr, Lindberg RB, McManus WF, Mason AD, Jr. Current approach to prevention and treatment of Pseudomonas aeruginosa infections in burned patients. *Rev Infect Dis* **55:**889-897, 1983.
15. Pruitt BA Jr, Mcmanus AT. Opportunistic infections in severely burned patients. *Amer J Med* **76:** 146-53; 1984.
16. Ramakrishnan KM *et al*. Incidence of burn wound sepsis in 600 burned patients treated in a developing country. Burns No. **11:** 404-407,1985.
17. Ramakrishnan KM *et al*. The management of anaerobic infection in extensive burns, Burns No. **12,** 270-72, 1986.
18. Robson MC, Heggers JP: Surgical infection. II. The β-hemolytic streptococcus. *J Surg Res* **9:**289-92,1969.
19. Solem LD, Zashe D, Strate RG: Ecthyma gangrenosum. Survival with individualized antibiotic therapy. *Arch Surg* **114:**580-583, 1979.
20. Teplitz C: The pathology of Burns and the fundamentals of burn wound sepsis in Burns - Team Approach Eds. Artz CP, Moncrief JA, Pruitt BA, W.B.Saunders .Co. Philadelphia 45-95, 1979.
21. Topley E *et al*: Assessment of red cell loss in the first two days after severe burns. *Ann Surg* **155:**581, 1962.
22. Zawacki BE: Reversal of capillary stasis and prevention of necrosis on burns. *Ann Surg* **180:**98, 1974.

PART II
Clinical Management

4

Initial Care of the Burn Wound

Burn injury occurs due to exposure to heat, chemicals, electricity or radiation. Depth and extent dictates the method of wound closure to be adopted. Acute burn wound management can be divided into three phases—namely the *Emergency phase*, which corresponds to the shock phase, and the *Acute Phase*, corresponding to the phase beginning with the cessation of emergency phase to the period when the burn wound completely heals. *Rehabilitation phase* corresponds to the period between wound healing and restoration of complete function.

EMERGENCY PHASE

Evaluation

The first step to be undertaken is the complete evaluation of the burn wound, with respect to the size, depth, age of the patient and nature of burn. Evaluation is further divided into primary and secondary surveys. In the primary survey, life-threatening problems like asphyxia are taken care of. Secondary survey deals more elaborately with the patient; assessing the extent of burn, depth, sites (special areas like the eyes) and charting of the area for calculation of the total body surface area burnt. Shock also should be identified because assessing the overall general condition of the patient certainly needs priority, before the burn wound is evaluated. Smoke inhalation injury and associated trauma, like head injuries and spinal cord injuries are taken care of first. Then the management of burn wound must be initiated.

Emergency Measures

Basic and simple measures are undertaken to protect the wound from the exterior environment. After removal of all burnt clothing, the patient is laid down on a clean sheet, and another one is used to cover the wound. A thorough questioning into the history of occurrence from the relatives or friends has to be documented. Reference to the way in which the burn occurred is very important in certain special burns like the smoke inhalation and the chemical burns, where urgent attention for systemic and local therapy have to be started. Patients who need immediate attention must be individualized and admitted into the intensive care unit. General measures that have to be undertaken in the initial wound care are described below:

Prevention of Occurrence of Further Damage

This is very important. Prevention is directed towards the cooling of the burnt surface, which still has high temperature in the burnt area, and secondly by irrigation and removal of caustic agents, which continue to damage the skin in the case of chemical burns.

Cooling

Copious amount of clean cold water can be applied by either sponges or directly on the burnt area. This procedure will bring down the extent of damage to the area in deep partial thickness burns. Pain also gets reduced when cold water is applied. One should be careful in using this procedure on the face. If water is poured inadvertently, the water may go into the nostrils, and get aspirated. The secretion of histamine by the mast cells gets reduced by cooling, and this will reduce the edema formation. The water used must be cool and not ice-cold. Icecold water or icepacks should not be used on extensive burns especially in children as this will cause severe hypothermia and further complicates resuscitation.

Neutralizing the Chemical Burns

All chemical burns must be washed with copious amounts of cold water. This will prevent desiccation of the skin. Judicious use of neutralizing agents, its advantages and disadvantages are described in the chapter on chemical burns.

But usually by the time the patient arrives in the emergency care ward, the burn would have cooled off by itself; therefore there is no place for cooling.

Hypothermia

Rapid cooling of a major burn used to be advocated in some countries, but hypothermia accelerates heat loss, and without proper monitoring, the patient may go into a sudden cardiovascular depression. This procedure is not adopted today. Every burn patient before cooling must have his core temperature assessed.

Pain Control

Soonafter sustaining burn, all patients suffer from intense pain. When the superficial epithelium gets peeled of, in a partial thickness burns, the burning pain is intense. The eschars formed in deep burns are devoid of pain sensation but when they crack or when dressing changes are done, these areas become very painful. The first line of pain medication is to give narcotics, and the preference is morphine. Small doses are administered intravenously. Subsequently, analgesics are supplemented. During dressing changes also, it is customary to use short acting analgesics like *Ketamine* and *Propofol.*

Cleaning the Wound

Wound is washed with tepid water and a solution of chlorhexidine or mild soap. Then the excess water is sponged of with cotton sponges **(Figure 4.1)**. Alternatively patients can be placed in a tub or under a shower to clean the wound **(Figure 4.2)**. Depending on the offending

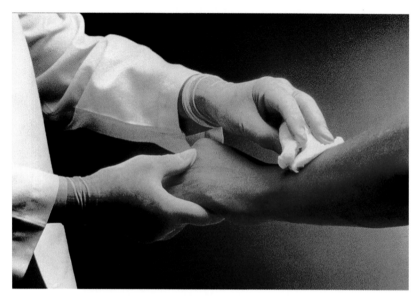

Figure 4.1: Initial washing and cleaning of a small partial thickness wound

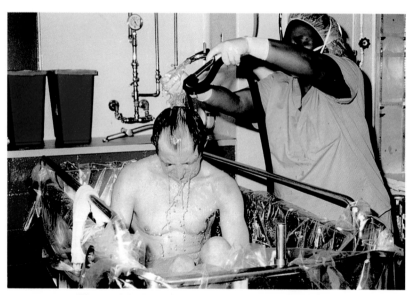

Figure 4.2: A combination of tubbing and shower being used to clean major burn wounds

agent that has caused the burn, washing the area is decided. In chemical burns, copious amount of cold water and normal saline are used to wash of the area. Neutralizing solution (alkalis for acids) are very judiciously used for fear of further damage to the burn. The neutralizing reaction in itself may further damage the area. Special solvent like mineral oil or

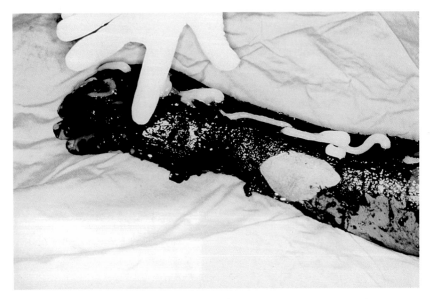

Figure 4.3: Tar burns of the upper extremity; application of
Petroleum based ointment to facilitate removal

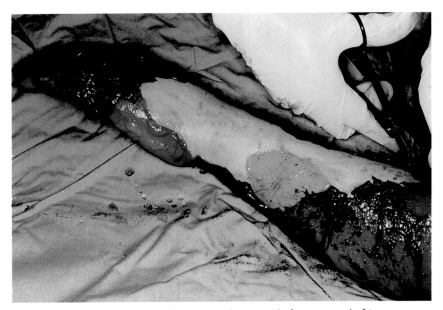

Figure 4.4: Same patient, wound exposed after removal of tar

petroleum based ointment must be used for removal of tar and asphalt burns, which have close structural affinity to these solutes. These solvents must be non-irritating, and non-toxic (Figures 4.3 and 4.4).

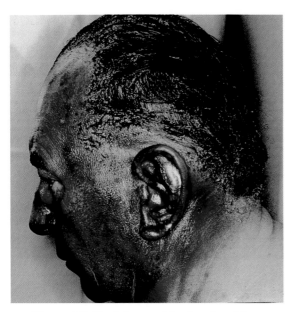

Figure 4.5: Flash burns of the head and face

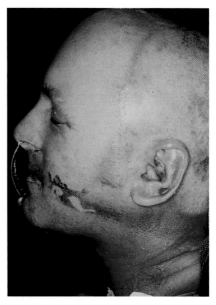

Figure 4.6: Same patient, exposed burn wound after shaving the scalp and cleaning the wounds

Hair bearing areas of the skin adjacent to the burn wounds should be shaved with at least one inch clear margin from the wound. The exception to this rule is eyebrow. Eyebrows should not be shaved and eye lashes should never be clipped **(Figures 4.5 and 4.6).**

Topical Agents

Many centers advocate the use of topical anti-microbial agents on the burnt surface after cleaning. For small superficial burns a soothening emollient like paraffin tulle gras will be comfortable to the patient when applied to the surface. If a physician wishes to use an antimicrobial agent, then 1% silver sulphadiazine is the best choice.

Dressing of the Wound

Dressings are used on burn wounds in the acute stage. As the wounds are very sensitive to the external air, they become very painful when exposed due to exposure of fine nerve terminals. Superficial burns and some hand burns feel more comfortable with dressings. Dressings have the following beneficial effects and are hence used regularly.

i. The wound is protected and the dressing prevents desiccation.
ii. It absorbs most of the exudates.
iii. Pain gets relieved to a greater extent.
iv. After eschar separate they are either removed or excised and the area left behind needs a dressing to prevent drying of the bed.
v. Dressings protect the grafted areas, and immobilize the grafts.

vi. Dressings also conserve body temperature by reducing evaporative water loss from the wound surface.

Dressings are of various kinds; they are: (a) Absorbent dressings, (b) Synthetic dressings, (c) Biological dressings. Biological dressings are described in greater detail in a separate chapter. Exudates are absorbed from the weeping wounds using absorbent dressings. Their thickness is gauged by the quantity of the exudates. A firm bandage is applied over the coarse mesh gauze pad dressing, in such a way that the blood circulation does not get impeded. Once crust formation begins to occur, absorbent dressings that become dry even if they are bulky will start irritating the area. In such an event, a thin layer of petrolatum gauze can be directly applied over the wound and dressed with coarse mesh gauze. Dressings are preferably changed once a day. Facial burns are not usually covered with any dressings, because it becomes very cumbersome to apply them.

Several semipermeable membrane dressings are available and are designed to provide a vapour and bacterial barrier and control pain while the underlying superficial wound or donor site re-epithelialises. There are single layer, and bilayered synthetic membranes.

Absorbents

These materials plug and conceal the exudates. These are the oldest class of dressings. Plant fibers such as linteum and oakum are used. Samson Gamgee created a tissue composite of fine jeweller's cotton wrapped in tiffany, the first absorbent pad designed that was based on the absorbent function of the woven fabric.

Impregnated Dressings

Dressings impregnated with an additive to create a non-adherent or semi-occlusive surface are available. Paraffin gauze developed during the World War I is the predecessor of various impregnated dressings. Petrolatum impregnated ones came later. Antibacterial incorporated in these nonadherent dressing materials are, framycetin, povidone-iodine, acemannan-aloe vera, and xeroform. A nonadherent impregnated dressing is often used as a primary dressing in superficial wounds **(Figure 4.7)**.

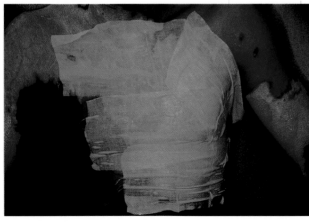

Figure 4.7: Healing of superficial partial thickness burns being dressed with petroleum based xeroform gauze dressing

Transparent Films

Adhesive films that are transparent, semipermeable, highly flexible and conforming to the contour of the surface provide relief from shearing forces. These dressings are used on partial thickness wounds. These contain polymers such as polyurethane, polyethylene, polycaprolactone, polytetrafluoroethylene, dimethyl aminoethyl methacrylate (Tegaderm, Dermafilm, Opsite, Oprafix etc). These are less popular.

Foams and Sprays

Foam dressings are sheets of foamed solutions of polymers such as polyvinyl alcohol, polyurethane, which are superior to film dressings in their providing thermal insulation and help to maintain moist environment at the wound surface. They are gas permeable, non-adherent, light and comfortable. They do not conform to the surface and cannot be used on certain anatomical sites.

Spray dressings are more comfortable to the wound surface. Most sprays are copolymers. Aeroplast is a copolymer of hydroxy-vinylchloride acetate modified maleic resin ester.

Composite Dressings

These are composed of laminates of two or more layers. The outer layer is durable and elastic and serves as water vapour control, the inner layer is adhesive. These dressings are hydrocolloids, hydrogel sheets, and gels.

Hydrocolloid dressings are compound formulations containing elastomeric adhesive and gelling agents. Carboxy methyl cellulose is the most common absorptive ingredient.

Epigard contains inner reticulated polyurethane and an outer polytetrafluoroethylene. Granuflex consists of outer polyurethane foam and an inner polymer / hydro-colloid complex.

Hydrogel sheets are 3-D network of cross linked hydrophilic polymers, such as polyethylene oxide, polyacrylamide and polyvinylpyrrolidine. An amorphous form where the polymer has not been cross linked is available which contain collagen, alginate or complex carbohydrates and have the ability to deliver moisture to a dry wound eschar and facilitate autolytic debridement in wounds.

Positioning the Patient after Dressings

This is also very important. Limb burns must be kept elevated, but in a comfortable way to the patient. Burn injury elicits edema in the tissues immediately adjacent to the wound. This makes the patient resent movement, and hold the limb in a dependent position. Hence elevation of parts is very important. For limb burns, in addition to elevation, ace bandages are also used to give gentle and uniform pressure and compression. This is combined with early physical rehabilitation.

Outpatient Burn Care

Small burn wounds and superficial burns are treated as out patient. The wounds are cleaned and if there is any history of contamination of the wound, the preference is to apply topical antimicrobials to prevent colonization of the wound. If the burns are small and superficial, they can be covered with wet saline dressings or petroleum based ointment. The wound usually heals in two weeks time. Pain also gets relieved in 24 hours time.

Superficial Partial Thickness

Burns which are devoid of epithelium can be covered with emollient dressings like paraffin tulle gras, and analgesics can be given. But if there are deeper areas in between the superficial partial thickness burns,then topical antimicrobials are indicated. Superficial partial thickness burns of the face often forms uncomfortable dry crusts and become painful. Hence it is better to use a thin layer of antimicrobial creams over the exposed burn surface. Some superficial partial thickness burns are of a weeping nature. These certainly require dressings. The oozing of the fluid is maximum soon after the injury. Over a layer of topical antimicrobial, thick gauze-pad dressings are applied and a firm bandage is applied. In the case of hand burns the fingers are all dressed separately, to facilitate active mobilization. The dressings are changed everyday, according to the level of soiling that occurs in the dressing. This is purely arbitrary and should be left to the individual needs of the patient and burn unit protocol.

Deep Burns

These have to be treated in a different way. To make them less susceptible to bacterial invasion, a thick film of topical antimicrobials are applied. The early removal of the totally devitalized skin and replace with autografting is the gold standard that one has to aim. But various factors like the availability of blood, donor sites and the general condition of the patient have to be considered carefully.

Burns of the Special Areas

Eye, hand and ear burns need early and definitive attention. Thorough evaluation of the part and proper documentation of the burnt area, according to the depth are necessary. For example in the eye burns, the appearance of the cornea, conjunctiva are first assessed; followed by the area of the lids. Prioritisation is according to the site of burn. The cornea gets the utmost priority in eye burns. The eyes are cleaned, irrigated preferably with normal saline and subjected to a thorough examination by the ophthalmologist.

Hand burns needs critical evaluation, and may need escharotomies, when vascular embarrassment is noticed.

Ear burns are assessed for cartilage damage and are nursed carefully and protected from pressure, or else cartilage necrosis, chondral abscess formation, and ultimate formation of a cauliflower like ear will be imminent.

Perineal burns also have to be carefully assessed, cleansed and the decision to place an indwelling catheter before edema sets in has to be thought of.

Place of Biological Dressings in Acute Burns

These dressings are very valuable and their use in acute burn wound management is described in the chapter on biological dressings. When autografts are sufficiently not available, one resorts to biosynthetic dressings and artificial skin after primary excision of the burn wound.

Management of Blister

There are two schools of thought as far as blister is concerned. Some believe that if left undisturbed the wound healing and epithelialization occurs much faster in a moist environment of the blister fluid. However, if multiple blisters are present they usually get punctured due to shearing movement and pressure. In such situations, keeping the blisters intact is not possible. The area of the punctured blisters may become a nidus for infection.

The second group of people thought that blister fluid is harmful, because it contains several harmful inflammatory mediators. The blister is not a closed wound as was once thought. It is their opinion to de-roof the blister and dress the area after cleaning. The authors recommend debridement of all blisters (Figures 4.8 and 4.9)

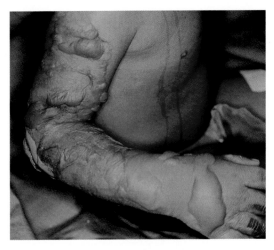 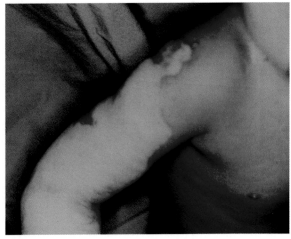

Figure 4.8: Intact and partially broken burn blisters on the upper extremity

Figure 4.9: Exposed partial thickness burns after debridement of all the blisters and cleaning of the wound in the same child

Burn Edema

Edema formation is rapid in the first three hours. The mechanism of edema formation has already been described in the previous chapter. To reduce the edema formation and to bring about anti-inflammatory response, pharmacological modulations are done. This is dealt with in detail in the chapter on pharmacological modulation of the burn wound. Commonly used drugs are steroids, enzymes; trypsin-chymotrypsin and Heparin. In deep burns, edema formation further reduces the quantum of Oxygen supplied per gram of tissue burnt, and thickness of necrosis increases. The depth of the wound is also an important predictor in burns with edema. Edema reaches maximum in 12 hours and in an uncomplicated wound resolves in 72 hours or longer. Certainly medications resolve it by reducing the pro-inflammatory cytokine IL6.

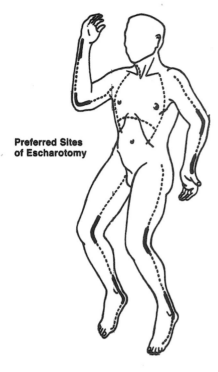

Preferred Sites of Escharotomy

Figure 4.10: Preferred sites of escharotomy on the chest, upper and lower extremities (Reproduced with kind permission from Lippincott Williams & Wilkins (formerly Little Brown & Company) Authors Takayoshi Matsuda and Marella Hanumadass. Editors Robert E Condon & Lloyd M Nyhus. "Manual of Surgical Therapeutics," 1996, Ninth Edition, Page 298, Chapter 17, Figure 2)

Eschar Management

In the acute phase of the burn wound, eschar is merely devitalized full thickness skin. If these eschars are constricting over any area, immediate escharotomies have to be done to prevent vascular embarrassment and compartmental syndrome. The escharotomies are done along the lateral axis of the limb and must go to the depth of the deep fascia. The veins on the surface of the deep fascia must be filled with unclotted blood. After doing the escharotomies, the peripheral pulse is checked and once the pulse has returned, a firm bandage is applied. Any bleeding points must be carefully cauterized, because there are occasions when significant blood loss might take place from the wound after escharotomy. Patient is usually given analgesics like propofol before embarking on the procedure. Commonly escharotomies are done in the limbs and chest wall **(Figures 4.10 to 4.13)**. Adequate replacement of fluids particularly Plasma must be given as escharotomy produces considerable loss of fluid and protein.

Management of Deep Burns in a Tertiary Care Facility in a Burn Center

Every deep burn that is admitted to the intensive care unit of a burn center requires special attention with regard to the burn wound.

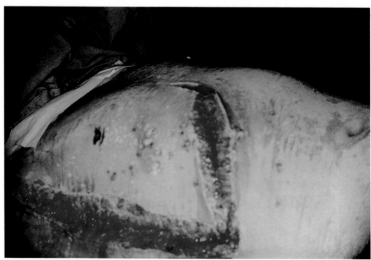

Figure 4.11: Escharotomy of the chest along the anterior axillary and subcostal lines

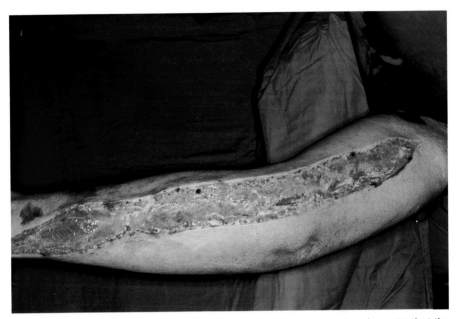

Figure 4.12: Escharotomy on the medial aspect of the upper extremity; note that the line of incision was placed anterior to the medial epicondyle to prevent injury to the ulnar nerve.

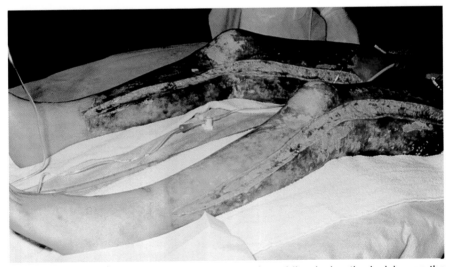

Figure 4.13: Escharotomy on the lower extremity; while placing the incision on the lateral aspect of the leg one should be careful not to injure the common Peroneal nerve as it lies on the neck of the fibula

The patient is made to lie down on a clean sheet after doing the initial debridement (removal of skin tags and de-roofing the blisters). The exposed areas are evaluated for any necessity for escharotomy. If need be, this is performed. The decision to treat the burn by exposure or with closed dressing is decided next. Once the patient is stabilized from the fury of shock, decision is taken with regard to excision of the burn wound either tangentially or full thickness (if the area of burn is small). The excised area is covered with split skin graft, obtained from the patient, or homograft from a donor or stored cadaver homograft. The details are given in the Chapter on Surgical Management of Burn Wounds. There are certain occasions, when primary reconstruction may have to be done when vital structures like major blood vessels, nerves or tendons are exposed; for example; in electrical injuries.

Definitive Burn Wound Care

This includes, daily cleaning of the burn wound, bath, dressings, and physical therapy. Superficial partial thickness burns are dressed daily till epithelialisation occurs by the end of 2nd week. Deep partial thickness wounds are watched daily for progress of wound healing. If the wound healing is satisfactory, one can wait. But if any areas are getting converted to deeper burn, then it is surgically excised and skingrafted. Grafted areas are also cleaned and dressed once in 4 days. When grafting has been done over the joints, the joint is immobilized to facilitate take of the graft.

BIBLIOGRAPHY

1. Burke JF, Bondoc CC, Quinby WC Jr, Remensnyder JP: Primary surgical management of the burned hand. *J Trauma* **16:** 593-98.
2. Demling RH, Mazes RB, Wolberg W: The effect of immediate and delayed cool immersion in burn edema formation and resorption. *J Trauma* **19:** 56-60, 1979.
3. Hartford CE: The bequests of Moncrief and Moyer: An appraisal of topical therapy of burns. American Burn Association Presidential Address 1981. *J Trauma* **21:** 827-834, 1981.
4. Haynes BWJ: Out patient Burns. *Clinics in Plastic Surgery* **1:** 645 -51, 1974.
5. Herndon DN: *Total Burn Care*; W.B. Saunders Co. 1997.
6. Ofeigsson OJ: Water cooling first aid treatment for scalds and burns. *Surgery* **57:**391-400, 1965.
7. Rockwell WB, Ehrlich HP: Should burn blister fluid be evacuated". *Burn care and Rehabilitation*; **11:** 93-95,1990.
8. Stratta RJ, Saffle JR, Kravitz M, Warden GD: Management of tar and asphalt injuries. *Am J Surg* **146:** 766-69,1983.
9. Waymack JP, Pruitt BA Jr: Burn wound care. *Adv Surg* **23:** 261-289,1990.

5

Topical Antimicrobial Therapy

The advent of effective topical therapy has been exciting and rewarding since the previous century. It is a unique example of a combined effort between the clinician and the laboratory scientist.

RATIONALE FOR USE

Burn wounds provide an excellent nidus for bacterial growth, particularly due to the fact that all the vascular channels are thrombosed. Initially thermal trauma coagulates the blood in the vessels and once the colonization occurs on the wound surface and the thrombosis progresses. Partial thickness wounds are thus converted to full thickness injuries.

In the absence of patent vascular channels systemically administered antibiotics, and cellular host defensive mechanism cannot reach the site of the burn. In such a situation, the only alternative is to use topical antimicrobial agents and this is the most logical approach.

Today it is understood that the major source of all the ill effects that is seen in the burn patient is due to the outcome of the burn wound. A combination of bacteria, which reside on the wound surface, first colonizes the burn wound. Among these bacteria, *Staphylococcus* predominates. Through hair follicles, these bacteria start invading the devitalized areas of burn. In 4 to 5 days the invasion gets established. Then gram-negative bacteria assumes a dominant role, particularly by *Pseudomonas aeruginosa*. By the end of the first week, well established invasive infection sets in. The topical antimicrobials are essentially used to prevent the spread of the bacteria beyond the burn wound. Hence, most often these are prophylactically used. But this action cannot be compared with the action of systemic antimicrobials. It is clearly understood that systemic antibiotics will not reach the dead tissue, and there is no advantage in using topical antimicrobials in an invasive burn wound sepsis, where organisms have entered the blood stream, causing septicemia.

In superficial partial thickness burns, also there is a place for topical antimicrobials. These help in controlling the colonization of bacteria, thereby preventing conversion of superficial partial thickness wounds into deeper burns. Therefore, if applied early; topical antimicrobials are chiefly chemoprophylactic in delaying colonization for prolonged periods. They are not chemotherapeutic, for established deep infections.

The ideal topical antimicrobial agent should have the following qualities:
A. Must be effective against broad spectrum of organisms, present in the burn wound, particularly the gram-negative rods.

B. Capable of active penetration of the wound in effective concentration, without any systemic toxicity.

C. Uninhibited by tissue fluids or bacterial products.

D. This agent if at all absorbed must be metabolized and excreted, in a short period.

E . Should not develop resistance. There is no topical agent available yet that satisfies all the above qualities.

The agents that are available are:

Silver Sulfadiazine

This is a substance synthesized by a reaction between silver nitrate with sodium sulfadiazine. This is available as a micronized water soluble cream with a strength of 1%. In this concentration, in-vitro studies the bacteria perish.

The exact mode of antimicrobial effect is still not definite. It is a well known competitive inhibitor of para-aminobenzic acid. It is suggested that silver sulfadiazine acts primarily on *bacterial* DNA replication.

Clinical trials have proved that it is a highly efficient prophylactic agent against gram-negative bacteria. In extensive burns, studies have proved that it delays colonization by gram negative bacteria for 10 to 14 days. Silver sulfadiazine has been widely used all over the world for the last many years. Currently, it is the gold standard for topical antimicrobial therapy for burn wounds. Many clinical trials have shown no bacterial resistance emerging after its use. Recently, protracted use of silver sulfadiazine has produced resistance to enterobactor species. The disadvantages are transient leukopenia, because some absorption of silver sulfadiazine takes place.

About 5% of patients have shown cutaneous hypersensitivity reactions. But these are not serious in nature.

It is easily applicable. One can liberally apply on the cleansed surface of the burn **(Figure 5.1)**. This can be left open as in exposure method of treatment, or can also be covered with a comfortable bulky bandage with minimal pressure **(Figure 5.2)**. Patients can have bath daily and the cream can be reapplied. In dressing extensive burn wounds, one can apply the cream on large gauze pads and lay over the wounds. Bandages can be applied to fix the dressings. If left undisturbed on a burn surface, layers of silver sulfadiazine with proteinaceous fluid exudates may form a pseudo - eschar.

SILVER NITRATE SOLUTION

0.5% solution in distilled water vehicle is applied every 2 hours with thick absorbent gauze dressings with bandages. An infusion bottle is used to store the solution, and the outlet tube, which is controlled with a devise, is inserted into the dressings, so that there will be a constant flow of the solution. Patients are nursed on disposable sterile draw sheets. Manually the dressings are changed twice in 24 hours. Some debridement of the wound occurs during the change of dressings. The effect of this agent is through "oligodynamic action". The active agent is minimally absorbed; absorbed silver has minimal toxicity if any.

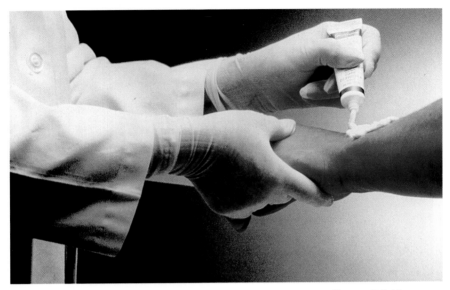

Figure 5.1: Silver sulfadiazine cream is directly applied to a small superficial burn wound

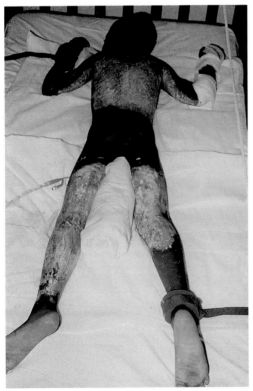

Figure 5.2: Burn wounds covered with silver sulfadiazine cream being treated by exposed method

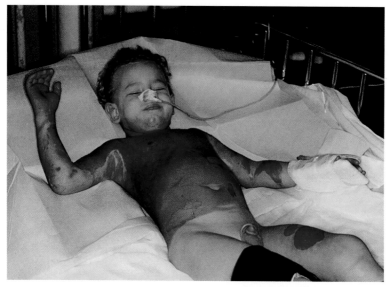

Figure 5.3: Deep burns in a 4 year old child

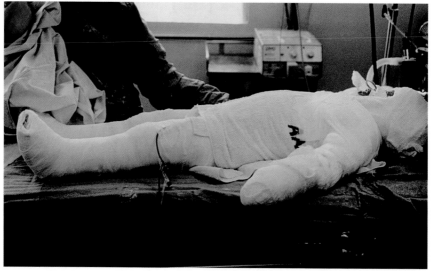

Figure 5.4: Early excision of the wound and skin grafting performed on the 3rd day. The remaining partial thickness burns, grafted areas and donor sites treated with 0.5% silver nitrate solution and bulky dressing

Prolonged contact with the wound results in absorption of large quantities of the vehicle, which is, distilled water resulting in concentration of silver nitrate. Concentrations of 1 to 2% can damage epithelial growth. Higher concentrations result in chemical injury and increase the depth of burn.

The combined effect of hypochloremia and hyponatremia, that develops can cause electrolyte imbalance particularly in children and in infants. Sometimes, counter therapy

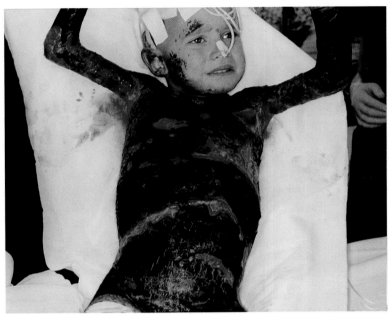

Figure 5.5: Same child two weeks after excision and grafting.
Grafts taken, but see the black discoloration of the grafts

with sodium chloride solution may have to be given either orally or intravenously (20 to 30 gms per day in adults) Another disadvantage is the staining of all objects that it comes into contact—Skin, clothes as well as the hands of nursing personnel **(Figures 5.3 to 5.5).**

The advantage is its effectiveness against wide spectrum of bacteria encountered. It is effective over recent grafts, donor sites and in preventing fungal infections. Resistance has also not been reported. But the whole procedure of dressing is very cumbersome, and it has almost come into disrepute.

Mafenide Acetate (Sulfamylon)

This sulfonamide - like drug is used as a 10% concentration in a water soluble cream base and is used to cover the burn wound as a thick cover, and is applied twice a day. The drug gets absorbed rapidly within 3 hours and is very effective in controlling bacterial population. The disadvantage is the occurrence of varying degrees of burning pain when applied in areas of partial thickness burns and the occurrence of maculopapular rash over unburned areas.

The biochemical effects of sulfamylon, is the strong carbonic anhydrase inhibiting property which results in impairment of the renal buffering mechanism, producing bicarbonate diuresis, and metabolic acidosis.

Recently 5% sulfamylon aqueous solution became popular. The osmolality of the solution is approximately 380m osm/L vs. 2,000 for sulfamylon cream. It is effective in combination with skin grafts, and biological dressings. It does not cause any metabolic derangement but, retains its potent antibacterial activity.

Gentamicin

Gentamicin is an aminoglycoside, and in 0.1% concentration in either ointment or cream base can be used over burn wounds. In a water soluble vehicle, it is supposed to release the drug effectively. The drug also gets absorbed systemically, and hence occlusive dressings cannot be used with gentamicin cream because, when it gets absorbed rapidly, during the interim phase between dressings, the burn wound is left unprotected.

The disadvantages are the accompanying ototoxicity on the 8th cranial nerve and nephrotoxicity. Rapid absorption of small quantities of the drug results in the emergence of resistant organisms.

The cream is very effective against *Staphylococcus* and *Streptococcus* and particularly against gram-negative rods, the *Pseudomonas* and the *E. coli*. Due to the toxicity its use as a topical antimicrobial agent is very limited today, and it should be reserved as a systemic chemotherapeutic drug for established gram-negative systemic infections.

Cerium Nitrate Silver Sulfadiazine

Cerium is one of the lanthanide elements and is supposed to have a large in-vitro antibacterial and antifungal spectrum. Cerium nitrate was combined with silver sulfadiazine as a water soluble cream, with sulfadiazine, a little less than 1%. This was used on burns as a thin cream and wounds were covered, with dressings. The precise mechanism of action of cerium is not known. It merely provides a potentially active antimicrobial substance in vivo. But the disadvantage is that when it comes into contact with burn wound fluid, it becomes inactive.

Though the initial results of this combination cream was applauded by some centers, today it is not known to be very useful, as resistant strains do develop when continuously used.

Framycetin Sulfate

As a 1% water soluble cream, is found to be a prophylactic topical agent, against most of the bacteria, particularly the *Staphylococcus*. As systemic absorption is very minimal and resistant strains have not emerged. There are no known serious toxic reactions, except rare cases of hypersensitivity. Exposure method of treatment with framycetin cream is possible.

Chlorhexidine and Povidone Iodine

Chlorhexidine conjugate is known to have a wide bacterial spectrum. But the application is painful. Resistance is unknown. For small burn wounds, povidone iodine cream can be used. When applied to a large burn wounds the iodine gets absorbed and can cause hepatic and renal dysfunction. Both these agents are of limited use.

Furacin (Nitrofurazone)

Furacin was first introduced during the second World War as a topical agent for surgical wounds, burns, chronically infected wounds and donor sites. It is bacteriocidal and acts by inhibiting the enzymes necessary for bacterial carbohydrate metabolism. Antimicrobial spectrum extends to both grampositive and gramnegative organisms. The advantages of furacin as a topical agent are that it penetrates rapidly through the eschar with minimal hypersensitivity. It has good grampositive coverage with low incidence of development of resistance. Its disadvantages are that it is not active against pseudomonas and causes, discomfort on application. The polyethylene glycol present in the base can exacerbate renal failure.

Currently, its use is reserved for the treatment of methecillim resistant staph aureus (MRSA) infections of the superficial burn wounds, skin grafted areas and donor sites.

Strategy for Topical Antimicrobial Therapy

A protocol should be designed in a burn unit, in the use of topical anti-microbial therapy, which includes:

a. Easy availability of large quantities of the cream must be ensured.

b. The cream that is used must be useful against the bacteria of prevalence in the unit.

c. The bacteria that is the common offending agent in the burn unit must be identified - either *Staphylococcus* or gramnegative rods.

d. The type of application that is to be adopted, as exposure of the wound with cream, or to be covered with closed dressings must be decided.

e. The topical agents can be alternated over a period of time. The cream either silver sulfadiazine, or framycetin is continuously used on all patients for a period of six months in the burn unit and later withdrawn for a period of three months, so as to prevent the development of resistance. After culturing the organisms and noting the sensitivity, the cream can be reintroduced into the unit.

f. Combination of creams, alternating in relays in the same patient can be used if the culture studies prove that the organisms are sensitive. But these combination therapies are not practical and usually not undertaken in large burn units.

BIBLIOGRAPHY

1. CL Fox, Monafo WW, Ayvazian UK *et al:* Topical chemotherapy of burns using cerium salts and silver sulphadiazine. *Surg Gynec Obstetr* **144:** 668-672: 1972.
2. Herndon DN: 'Treatment of Infections' in *Total Burn care* chap. 11,123, W.B. Saunders Co. Ltd.
3. Monafo WW, Vatche H Ayuvazian. Topical Therapy" in *The Surgical Clinics of North America,* **58(6),** 1978.
4. Moncrief JA, Teplitz C: Changing concepts in burn sepsis. *J Trauma* 233-245,1964.
5. Moncrief JA: Topical therapy of the burn wound, Present status. *Clin Pharm Therapy* 10:439, 1969.
6. Moncrief LA: Topical antimicrobial therapy of the burn wound. *Clin Plast Surg* 1:563-576,1974.
7. Moyer CA, Bretano L, Gravens DI *et al:* Treatment of large human burns with 0.5% silver nitrate solution. *Arch Surg* **90:** 812-867,1965.
8. Pietsch J, Meakins JL: Complications of povidone iodine absorption in topically treated burn patients. *Lancet* 280-282,1976.
9. Ramakrishnan and Hanumadass, "Handbook of Burn Management", Jaypee Brothers Medical Publishers, India, 98-118, 1991 .
10. Shuck JM, Moncrief JA, Monafo WW: The management of burns. General considerations and the sulfamylon method, II: The silver nitrate method. *Current Probl Surg* Feb 1969.
11. Snelling CFT, Ronald AR, Waters WR *et al:* Comparison of silver sulfadiazine and gentamycin for topical prophylaxis against burn wound sepsis. *Can Med Assn Journal* **119:** 466,1978.

6

Biological Dressings and Skin Substitutes

Various types of wounds with different healing patterns have resulted in the preparation of a variety of wound coverings. Optimal environment is required for wound healing and the dressings maintain such an environment till the wound heals. Hence an ideal dressing material maintains a moist environment, acts as a bacterial barrier, is a medium for free exchange of gases, and provides a barrier against toxic contaminants. The ultimate goal in the management of the burn wound is to obtain physiological closure in the shortest period of time. The cover that is provided to achieve this must be durable and permanent. Autogenous skingraft remains the primary method of wound closure and is the gold standard for burn wound coverage. The paucity of available donor sites in extensive burns provided the impetus to look for materials that would provide temporary wound closure. During the past three decades, the use of biological and biosynthetic materials for the temporary closure of the wound has become common place. The biological dressings and skin substitutes have evolved based on the provision of such an ideal environment. Permanent skin substitutes include cultured epidermal grafts, acellular dermal matrix and composite dermal-epidermal grafts. (Classification: See Chart 6.1).

Inspite of the advances for the past two decades in the development of skin substitutes, autologous split thickness skingraft closure remains the standard of treatment for the full thickness and deep burn wounds. One should aim at achieving this physiological permanent closure as early as possible after the burning.

If the burns are too extensive with limited donor site, then one should consider utilizing the temporary skin substitutes. Apart from human cadaver homografts, biological temporary wound coverings include porcine xenograft, embryonic membranes from human and bovine sources, collagen membranes, reconstituted collagen from bovine and other sources like, embryo-foetus and neonatal skin. Biological dressings are derived from natural tissues consisting of various formulations and combinations of collagen, elastin and lipid. The biological dressings are far superior to the synthetic dressings. These restore water barrier and prevent dehydration of the wound, decrease the evaporative heat loss, protein and electrolyte loss in the exudate, prevent bacterial contamination, and improve the quality of healing.

BASIC DEFINITIONS OF BIOLOGICAL WOUND COVERINGS

A. Autograft: A graft which is transferred from one location to another on the same individual.

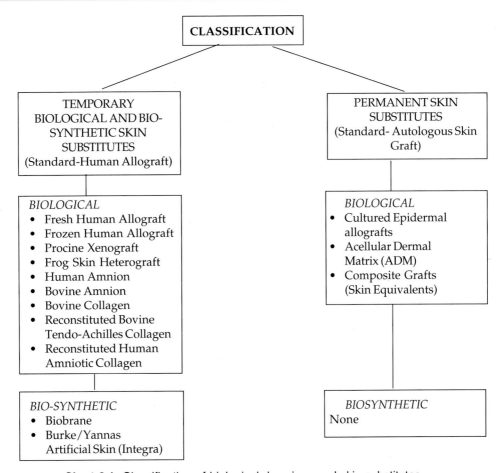

Chart 6.1: Classification of biological dressings and skin substitutes

B. Allograft: A graft which is transferred between two individuals of the same species (also known as homograft).
C. Heterograft: A graft transferred between individuals of different species

AUTOGENOUS SKINGRAFTS

Autologous skingrafts are indicated as a permanent coverage or replacement in full thickness burns and in deep partial thickness injuries. These grafts can be;
A. Split thickness skingraft (STSG): Epithelium and partial thickness of dermis; donor site heals by epthelialization and contraction.
B. Full thickness skingrafts (FTSG): Epithelium and full thickness dermis; including hair and sweat glands; donor site heals by primary closure or STSG. Full thickness skingrafts work best on a flat surface that is muscle or fascia and less on fat. The lack of "drape-ability" makes it less than ideal for irregular surface.

The choice of donor site depends on the size of the defect and quality of skin coverage desired. Split thickness skingraft heals with thin shiny surface, but has a better chance of "take" on a marginal recipient bed like fresh granulation tissue or freshly excised wounds. These thin grafts tend to contract. Full thickness skingrafts heal with better texture and color, may transfer hair, sweat glands and nerve endings with less contraction. These grafts are only available for small wound defects and are not practical for burn wounds. Split thickness skingrafts are the most common type of grafts for wound coverage of acute thermal injuries. A multitude of factors determines the choice of donor site location; thickness of the grafts and whether the skin should be meshed or sheet graft used . The thicker the graft the better the cosmetic appearance, color and less contracture. The epidermis is thinnest in infants, thickest at puberty and becomes thinner with increasing age. The dermis reaches maximum thickness about the 4th decade and then becomes thinner as age increases. Skin thickness varies from one anatomic area to another, i.e., very thin on the back of the hand, inner aspect of both the upper arms and thighs. The posterior trunk, especially the back and buttock, is an ideal donor site because of the very thick dermis. Repeat harvesting from the same donor is often a necessity, but with each harvest, reepithelialization takes longer. Donor site harvest in some anatomic areas is often difficult because there is little subcutaneous tissue. Techniques to improve procurement include injecting soft tissue with Ringer's lactate (RL), using towel clips to pull the skin, or applying pressure by squeezing the surrounding soft tissue. The color match is important. The closer the recipient site is to the donor, the better the color match. When grafting the face the donor site above the nipple- blush line gives better color matching; this includes the scalp. Donor sites in the elderly are best taken where the dermis is thickest.

Mesh vs Sheet Graft

Both the size of burn requiring grafting and the available donor sites are considerations as to whether to use sheet or mesh graft. A ratio of 1 : 1.5 results in almost no expansion and very minimal epithelization between the skin lattices. The greater the mesh ratio the thinner the split thickness, that needs to be harvested. This only reflects on the large size of the burn. Mesh graft conforms well to irregular contours. Either non expanded 1 : 1 or 1 : 1.5 results in equal functional outcomes as sheets, although, the cosmetic appearance is not as good as sheet grafts. The split thickness skingraft can be harvested with a free hand skin harvesting knife or a power dermatome (Figure 6.1).

Donor site preparation may mean nothing more than setting the dermatome to the desired thickness or adjusting the free hand knife before harvesting the skin. Depending on the width, length and location chosen, one may need to inject RL into the underlying subcutaneous tissue. Blood loss associated with harvesting increases with increasing thickness of the graft. A STSG measuring 4" x 8" is associated with a mean blood loss of 46 cc's. To decrease blood loss, especially when large donor areas are to be harvested, a vasopressor such as epinephrine (5mg/L saline) or neosynephrine (16 mg/1000cc RL) is added and gauze pads soaked in this solution are applied immediately to the harvested areas as pressure compresses. Neosynephrine is preferred because it has minimal arrhythmic potential.

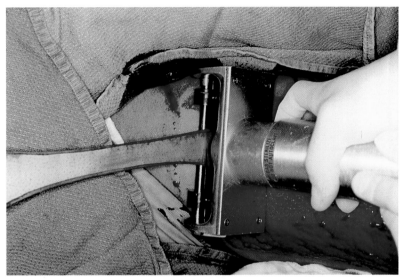

Figure 6.1: Split thickness skingraft being harvested with padget electric dermatone

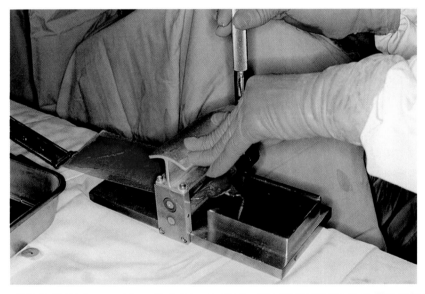

Figure 6.2: Split thickness skingrafts being meshed using Tanner's Mesher. The ratio of the meshed skin can be adjusted utilizing disposable plastic carriers of different ratio

The use of widely meshed skin is frequently necessary. The procedure of meshing skin should be simple and fast. There are several meshers available in the market **(Figures 6.2 and 6.3)**. Important factors imparting on a successful graft " take" includes : 1. Suitable graft bed; 2. apposition of the graft to the recipient site; 3. immobilization.

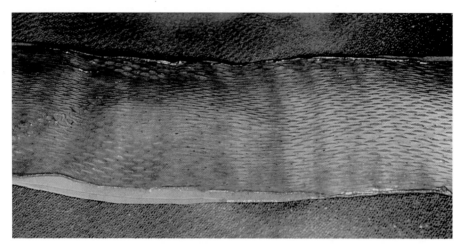

Figure 6.3: 1:1.5 ratio meshed skin was placed on thick moist sterile brown paper with dermal side up for easy placement of graft on the wound

Wound Bed

Nonviable tissue remains if inadequate excision of eschar is done; this may occur because if excision of a deep dermal burn is done too early, it may not be possible to accurately identify viable from nonviable bed. Other reasons include, the wound becoming bloody and obscuring non-bleeding area, and a lack of surgical experience. Absolute hemostasis is essential. Grafting on granulating wound bed requires scrapping or excision of granulation tissue. Skingraft will not "take" on avascular recipient bed, e.q. not over bare bone or tendon. Adipose tissue is suitable if the wound is fresh after surgical excision.

Infection

The local concentration of microbes is important. While major graft loss secondary to burn wound sepsis is now rare, local wound infection represents a problem. It is no longer common practice to routinely culture the wound prior to early excision and skingrafting. Qualitative cultures of full-thickness burns without histological evaluation are associated with inadequate information. Shuck determined the bacterial counts on recipient sites treated with homograft. When the bacterial count was <10 organisms per gram of tissue, autograft "take" was good. This method is objective, but infrequently utilized. Instead the surgeon will subjectively assess the quality of the recipient bed and determine if autografting is likely to succeed or not. Early excision prior to bacterial colonization is associated with high graft "take". Old granulating wounds should always be cultured and offending organisms should be excluded or treated before contemplating on grafting.

Movement of the Graft

Prevention of graft movement is of paramount importance in achieving successful autografting. Immobilization is generally not a significant problem when the recipient site is not over or adjacent to joints or areas associated with movement such as, face, neck, and buttocks.

Mesh graft will always have a "Crocodile-Like" appearance. The use of sheet graft has been promoted in pediatric burns. If sufficient donor sites are available one should consider their use. Their true advantage is cosmetic. Sheet graft requires constant attention so as to remove blood or serum. Although, Pie-Crusting the sheet will theoretically allow serum and blood to escape from under the graft, for all practical purposes this often does not happen. Once clot forms, it remains there. Many high volume burn units do not have the luxury of ample personnel to attend to this problem; therefore do not find the routine use of sheet grafts practical. Stent or Tie - Over dressing is an effective way to assure good apposition and at the same time provide for hemostasis.

Revascularization of the skingraft begins about the third day and is completed in a week. Fibrinous adhesion of skingraft to the recipient site enables one to remove a dressing after 72 hours. Granulation tissue initiates the process of wound contraction. An ungrafted wound bed contracts more than a grafted one. It appears that the force of contraction is not secondary to the graft but to the recipient bed. Granulation tissue will be reabsorbed under a skingraft and this may explain in part why contraction is less even with a very thin split thickness skingraft as compared to a wound allowed to heal without a graft.

Securing Grafts

Attachment of sheet or mesh graft is done without staples or sutures on the hand and digits. In extremities also where circumferential bandages can be applied, no fixation is generally required. Whenever sutures are used, 3-0 or 4-0 plain catgut or synthetic absorbable sutures are utilized. This is important in children. If nonabsorbable sutures are used, nylon is preferred to silk because it does not "drag" through the tissue. Because of their ease and speed of application, staples have for the most part replaced sutures. Occassionally, staples become "buried" and cause pain, local sepsis, or draining sinus. Absorbable staples made a brief appearance on the market. We believe there is a need for absorbable staples especially for the pediatric patient. Fibrin glue can be used to secure a skingraft. The cost and the time necessary to prepare it are modest drawbacks. Adhesive strips are a good way to secure grafts on the fingers and hand, and recommended in pediatric patients.

Dressings

Various authors have discussed which is most important for a good "take", pressure or immobilization. A variety of dressings can be used to cover grafts. These include a multitude of commercially available products and all seem to work well. There are certain problems inherent in the use of mesh graft which must be addressed in order to maximize the "take". Widely meshed skin covers very little of the recipient bed, consequently some type of wound coverage, whether a physiologic dressing (homograft, meshed or not meshed, or heterograft), or a synthetic dressing is recommended. Because of the cost and added operating room time associated with the application of multiple sheets of homograft, a Biosynthetic dressing like Biobrane is preferred. It has a number of benefits; transparent, stretches, and can be rapidly applied. It nevertheless may become very adherent to the open wound because of capillary ingrowth in the interstices. In some occasions, epithelization may be prevented. If the mesh expansion appears static, the dressing must be removed.

Several simple and inexpensive dressings include, petroleum based gauze, stent, foam pads, gauze rolls, fluffed gauze, cotton balls impregnated with mineral oil and wrapped inside of a piece of gauze. The dressing remains oily and doesn't stick to the skin when removed. A dressing of fine mesh gauze impregnated with an antibiotic will dry out and the graft will stick when the dressing is removed. More elaborate dressing techniques such as "quilt", first described by McGregor, are used. Quilting is used on large surface areas such as chest, abdomen, and back of the trunk.

HUMAN CADAVER HOMOGRAFT

Homograft from other human is often used as temporary wound cover in excised burn wounds. This temporary cover promotes wound vascularisation and prepares the wound bed which accepts an autograft after the removal of homograft. The first clinical use of allograft for the burn wound closure was recorded in 1881 by Gurdner, but modern era of allograft used as a biological dressing in extensive burns was popularized by Brown and Fryer in 1953.

Human allograft skin can be harvested from a live donor or from a human cadaver within twenty four hours after death, if the body is refrigerated. Because of the scarring of the donor sites and surgical morbidity, harvesting from live donor has been abandoned nowdays. The harvested skin can be used fresh or refrigerated at 4°C and is good for two weeks. Human skingraft can be preserved frozen (cryopreserved) in citrated plasma, or glycerol at - 70°C for an extended period. Successful take of these grafts results after thawing and grafting on a freshly excised wound with viable bed (Figures 6.4A to D).

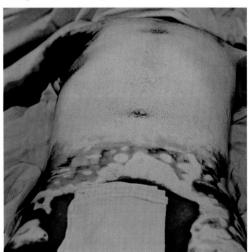

Figure 6.4A: Mixed full thickness and deep partial thickness burns of the anterior trunk

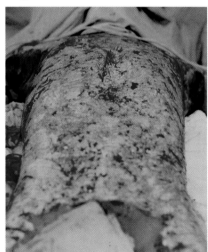

Figure 6.4B: Same patient; burn wounds excised sequentially upto the viable healthy tissue on the 3rd post-burn day

(Figures 6.4A to D Reproduced with kind permission from Dr. Thatte, Editor of the "Indian Journal of Plastic Surgery," December 1988. Volume 21. No. 2: "Recent Trends in Management of Burns" by Marella L. Hanumadass, Page 81, Fig. 10-13)

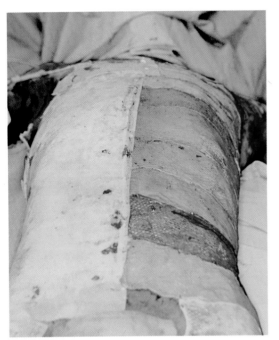

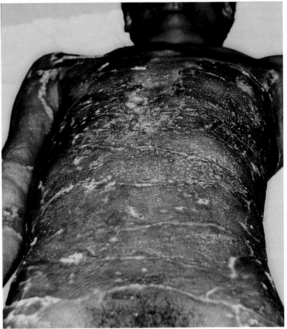

Figure 6.4C: The excised wounds covered with homografts over the left half of the trunk and biobrane on the right side, after achieving complete hemostasis

Figure 6.4D: After 10 days, homograft and biobrane were removed and replaced with split thickness meshed autografts. The picture shows the appearance of the autografts two weeks after surgery

Based on this experience human cadaver skin banks were established in the United States and Europe for later use. The homograft under optimal conditions vascularises and "takes" like patient's own skin until it gets rejected in two to three weeks or it is removed surgically prior to autografting.

The advantage of using the homograft is that it reduces water, electrolytes, and protein losses from the wound. It prevents the desiccation of viable tissue on the wound bed, suppresses bacterial proliferation and prepares the wound for definitive wound closure. With wound closed physiologically a reduction in energy requirement and pain is achieved. In recent times, it is also used to provide a dermal template for cultured epidermal grafts. Homograft is indicated for use in burn management for coverage of extensive wounds where autologous tissue is not immediately available or for the coverage of widely meshed skin autografts. They also can be used on wounds where autograft is not expected to take because of bacterial contamination or questionable viability of the wound bed.

The main disadvantages are the potential lack of availability, potential infectious disease transmission, antigenicity and rejection.

PORCINE SKIN HETEROGRAFT

Porcine skin has been widely used as temporary wound cover. Porcine cutaneous xenografts are readily available through the commercial production in western countries, which have satisfied the requirements of supply and demand. They are available in three forms: Fresh refrigerated, frozen or liophylized. The sterility is maintained by irradiation or antibiotic exposure, followed by chemical rinses and storage.

The evaluation of porcine skin as a biological dressing was pioneered by Bromerg and Song in 1965. Several laboratory and clinical studies demonstrated no vascularization of these grafts when placed on healthy granulation tissue or on excised wounds. Though the granulation tissue containing capillaries did penetrate xenograft dermis, no inosculation with porcine capillaries was observed.

It is, therefore, believed that porcine xenograft behaves only as a "dressing" when placed in contact with granulating wounds. No clinically significant evidence has been reported indicating of a major immune reaction between graft and host although detection of the humoral antibodies has been detected. While the exact nature of the immune response to split thickness cutaneous xenograft is yet to be determined, the clinical benefits derived from the use of porcine skin as a temporary biological dressing has been widely appreciated at burn units throughout the world.

Porcine skingrafts may be applied to any denuded wound surface after the major portion of devitalized tissue has been removed **(Figure 6.5)**. Because vascularization and classic rejection do not occur, grafts may be left in place 5-7 days or more, provided no subgraft suppuration develops due to residual necrotic debris. Wounds should be inspected daily and xenograft changed if adherence is not adequate due to suppuration. Unexplained temperature elevation may occur in certain instances, probably due to foreign protein reaction. Discontinuation of the use of porcine skin corrects this problem.

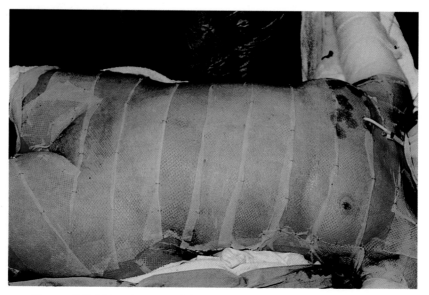

Figure 6.5: Extensive superficial partial thickness burns covered with meshed split thickness xenograft (porcine skin)

FROG SKIN HETEROGRAFT

The use of frog skin as a temporary biological dressing was reported by Piccolo *et al* from Brazil in 1992. In South America and Brazil where large sized frogs are available, the skin is harvested and the frog skin serves as a temporary biological cover for burn wounds in preparation for autografting. The advantage of frog skin is that it is non-antigenic, thin and easy to use.

AMNIOTIC MEMBRANE

The source of the amnion can be human or bovine. Large sheets of amnion can be harvested from bovine source. These are very thin and transparent and can be used to apply over large areas of burn wound. The role of amniotic membrane in covering partial thickness burn wounds has been well established ever since J.Pigeon (1960) made use of it. Its effective reduction of bacterial count in infected burn wounds was shown by Robson and Krizek (1973) and in contaminated granulation tissue by Bade (1958). It is quite effective due to its covering effect (Morris *et al* 1966) and due to the presence of Lysozyme, Oestrogen and Progesterone (Glask and Snyder 1970). Amniotic membrane alleviates pain, promotes epithelialisation and is also economical (Thompson and Parks 1981; Haberal *et al*, 1987). Amniotic membrane as an effective burn wound cover for partial thickness burns as has been convincingly noted by Pigeon J(1960), Dino *et al* (1966), Golocco *et al* (1974), Bose (1979), Piserchia and Akenzua (1981), Viswanath Rao and Chandrasekaran (1981), Ramakrishnan and Rao (1983), Ramakrishnan *et al* (1995).

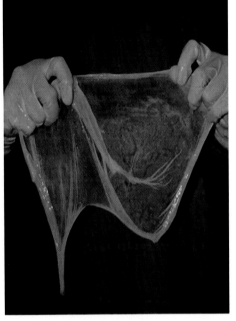

Figure 6.6: Amniotic membrane obtained at the time of cesarean section from a mother who is seronegative for HIV and HbSAg

Human amniotic membrane is separated from placenta obtained fresh from seronegative mothers with no history of premature rupture of membranes, or of infection with HIV, HbSAg and are used as biological covers. The membranes are cleaned in normal saline, the cotyledons are removed, rinsed and stored in 0.25 percent sodium hypochlorite solution at - 30°C to -90°C in a deep freezer for any length of time. But for immediate use, the harvested membrane is treated with gentamycin solution and is directly applied on burn wounds. It is very thin; easily adherent, easy to spread, conforms to all the contours of the body, reduces pain on application, and provides a moist environment underneath for epithelialisation.

Amniotic membrane is derived from the ectoderm. Amniotic membrane has a basement membrane similar to the one in the wound bed. It consists of type IV collagen, which is essential in healing wounds. The membrane is transparent and has many pores; through which exudation of discharge can take place **(Figure 6.6)**.

Method of Application

The burn wound is cleaned well, all dead skin is removed, exposing the live epithelial layer and the membrane is applied under sterile conditions, spreading a little over the adjoining intact skin, and allowed to adhere. Once the epithelialisation is complete, the membrane separates by itself from the sides and the healed wound gets exposed **(Figures 6.7A to C)**.

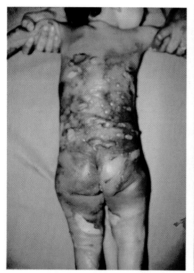 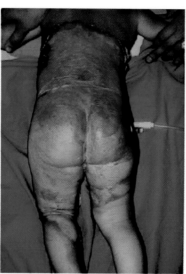 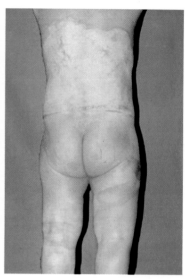

Figure 6.7A: Superficial partial and deep partial thickness burns in a 2 year old child due to scalding of the entire back, buttocks and thighs

Figure 6.7B: The same child after application of native amniotic membrane on the 4th day post burn

Figure 6.7C: The healed wound after 4 weeks showing complete epithelialization. The membrane was removed and reapplied twice at 10 day intervals

Uses of Amniotic Membrane Dressings

Earlier, amniotic membrane was used over contaminated wound surfaces and was found that the colony count decreased considerably. Also the amnion and the chorion layers were not separated initially. Later, amnion when separated was found to be very thin and transparent and was advantageous as a temporary wound cover. This thin amnion was often used on superficial partial thickness burn wounds and it is advantageous to use on deep partial thickness burn wounds also in that it prevents infection and bacterial colonization. Once the deeper burn area is dry, the Eschar along with the amnion is excised and autograft is applied. In larger burn area, when the areas after excision is not suitable for skingrafting, the excised area is covered with amniotic membrane again and this prepares the wound ideally for skingrafting.

Later the membrane is removed and autografting is done. Instances where repeated application of membrane and healing of the wound without skingrafting has been noticed, which is an advantage with amnion dressings.

Advantage of Amniotic Membrane as a Wound Cover

The following advantages of amniotic membrane as a wound cover are noted:
1. Amnion, when separated is very thin, transparent compared to other wound covers
2. It is easy to handle the amnion and it is flexible.
3. Amnion is easy to apply, spreads easily and can be used without hurting the patient.
4. Adherence of the membrane to the wound surface is very good and due to its porosity drainage of fluid also takes place.
5. Under the amnion dressing, one could visualize the progress of wound healing, due to its transparency.
6. Pain is much less after the application of the membrane.
7. The large quantity of estrogen, progesterone in the membrane also hastens epithelialisation.
8. When heparin was used as a spray over the burn wound covered with membrane, the healed scar was very satisfactory due to early collagen remodeling. It is easy to combine pharmacological agents like heparin and silver sulphadiazine with the membrane.
9. The cost of burn management and duration of hospital stay was considerably reduced, which is a great advantage in developing countries.
10. In a developing country with large incidence of burns like in India, amniotic membrane is very useful as a temporary biological dressing.

Disadvantages of Amniotic Membrane Dressings

a. Separation, preparation and storage of amniotic membrane dressings are little cumbersome, and labor intensive.
b. After the incidence of HIV infections, use of human tissues is under circumspect, even if all the precautions are taken.
c. Inadvertent use could infect the wound, if proper culture studies on the stored membrane are not done.

COLLAGEN

It is an insoluble fibrous protein of vertebrates that is the chief constituent of the fibrils of connective tissue (as in skin and tendons) and the organic substance of bones and yields gelatin and glue on prolonged heating with water. Collagen is found in the extracellular matrix. 20 types of collagen have been described till recently. Twenty five to 35% of body protein is collagen. Type I and Type III are more commonly seen in all the tissues. Commercially, collagen is extracted from bovine source; sheep's intestine, tendo-achilles of sheep and from the dermis.

Structure of Collagen

Collagen molecule is a rigid rod 2900 A° by 15 A° size triple helix in structure with 3 amino acids GLY-X-Y sequence repeated and glycine with a single carbon atom is in every 3rd residue and fits into the superhelix. It is stabilized by proline and hydroxyproline residues.

Functions of Collagen

Collagen has high content of diamino dicarboxylic amino acids and carbohydrate moieties, which makes it hydrophilic and very suitable for cell adhesion. Presence of glycoprotein like fibronectin promotes attraction of fibrogenic cells to collagen implants.Collagen gives strength and structure to the tissues, support to the hard tissues like bone, form and integrity to soft tissues, provides stiff layer to vessel wall, thus preventing its bursting, and degrades in the biological environment. It has low antigenicity, supports cellular growth. It has hemostatic properties. Collagen is commercially manufactured and is readily available for use. Dried collagen sheet is available, but this is not as efficient as preserved collagen.

Application of Collagen Sheet

The method of application of collagen sheet in the native form, from the bovine intestine is the same as it is for amniotic membrane. The wound is cleansed with antiseptic solution and covered with the collagen sheet after rinsing the sheet several times in normal saline and is allowed to adhere over a period of few hours. Collagen sheets are useful in the management of superficial partial thickness burns, and in deep partial thickness wounds **(Figures 6.8A to C)**. Collagen sheets are little thicker than the other membrane dressings and takes more time to spread on the wound. Collagen has all the properties of an ideal substitute and is used freely on open wounds.

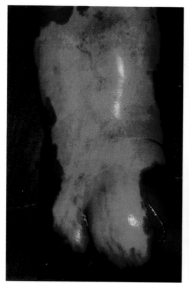 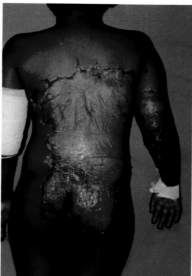 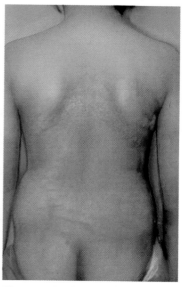

Figure 6.8A: 12 years old girl with superficial partial thickness burns of the posterior trunk and upper limbs

Figure 6.8B: The appearance of the wound on the 7th day after application of collagen membrane dressing

Figure 6.8C: Twenty five days after burn injury and removal of the collagen membrane, showing complete healing

RECONSTITUTED COLLAGEN

The Collagen is solubilized and purified and then attempts are made to reform and repolymerize the material in proper shape, and thus the Collagen is reconstituted in the form of a thin film. During the process of reformation and repolymerization, drugs can be incorporated and used for delivery to the wound surface. Both Human and Bovine collagen can be reconstituted **(Figures 6.9A to C).**

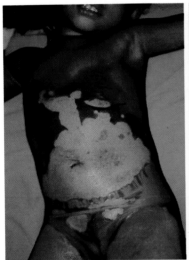 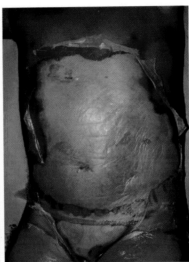 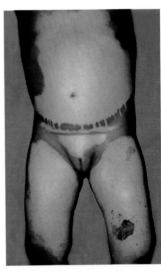

Figure 6.9A: 8 years old girl with superficial partial thickness burns anterior trunk and thighs first post burn day

Figure 6.9B: Appearance of the wound 6th post burn day after application of reconstituted amniotic collagen membrane

Figure 6.9C: Appearance of the wound after removal of reconstituted amniotic collagen membrane on the 14th day, showing complete healing

BIOSYNTHETIC SKIN SUBSTITUTES: BIOBRANE

Biobrane is a bilaminate membrane composed of a nylon mesh fabric bonded to an ultra thin layer or silicone rubber. The nylon fabric is coated with porcine peptides prepared from type I collagen, which are reported to facilitate adherence to the wound bed and promote fibrovascular ingrowth. To date it is the most successful biosynthetic dressing developed for general use in the care of burn injuries **(Figures 6.10 and 6.11).**

The silicone layer is semipermeable and allows passage of water vapor from the wound, while protecting the wound from external bacterial contamination. Studies have shown that when biobrane is applied over full-thickness wounds, vascular and connective tissue ingrowth occurs rapidly in 72 hours and adherence is equal to that of homograft until 10 days.

Biobrane is indicated for: (a) Temporary closure of the excised, full-thickness burn wounds prior to autograft placement. (b) Coverage of superficial partial-thickness burns until re-epithelialzation occurs. (c) Some burn units in the United States have used this material for dressing the donor sites. Biobrane is very expensive and has no significant advantage over simple non-adherent dressing over the donor sites. Its use for donor sites is not justified.

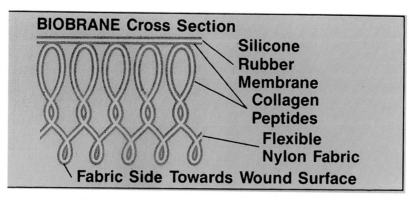

Figure 6.10: Cross-section diagram of biobrane

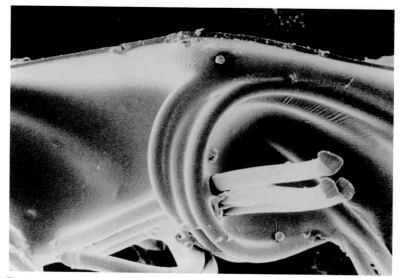

Figure 6.11: Electron microscopic cross-section appearance of biobrane. Silicone membrane layer on the top and nylon fabric coated with porcine collagen peptides underneath

Biobrane is contraindicated on wound with gross purulence or colonized wounds with microbial count greater that 100,000 organisms/ gram of tissue. Biobrane cannot be placed over any residual devitalized tissue on either full or partial-thickness wounds.

Method of Application

Superficial, partial thickness burns   Application should occur early after injury before microbial colonization occurs. Burn wound is cleaned and debrided of any obvious devitalized epithelium. Wounds are then covered with biobrane; which is secured in place to either itself or to the surrounding unburned skin with tape or steri strips. Slight stretching of the biobrane will facilitate contact with the wound surface. A light outer dressing may be employed for

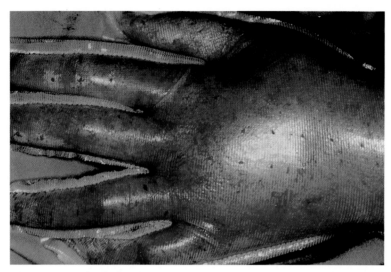

Figure 6.12: Superficial partial thickness burns on dorsum of the hand covered with biobrane glove. The wound can be observed through transparent membrane. The hand and fingers can be exercised without the restriction of a bulky dressing

protection and wounds observed for adherence and fluid collection (Figure 6.12). Biobrane will subsequently separate from the healed wound with minimal effort.

Excised full-thickness wounds The wounds should be excised to the level of viable tissue. Complete hemostasis is absolutely necessary before application of biobrane. It is secured with staples or sutures with slight tension to facilitate contact with the wound (Figures 6.4A to D). Wound should be observed for adherence and fluid collection under the Biobrane. Biobrane removed and autografts applied when donor sites are available and patient's condition permit.

BURKE/YANNAS ARTIFICIAL SKIN (INTEGRA)

In 1981, Burke and Yannas published preliminary clinical results of the use of the "Artificial Skin" they have developed as a wound cover. Since then it is the subject of extensive investigation. It is a bilayered biodegradable membrane; the dermal analogue is an open lattice of fibers made of bovine collagen, covalently linked to chondroitin 6 sulfate. The temporary outer layer, the epidermal component is a medical grade silicone 100 um thick. The artificial skin acts as a structured dermal regeneration template (Figure 6.13). When placed on an excised wound the dermal components becomes adherent and the epidermal component, silicone membrane protects the wound from desiccation and bacterial contamination. The artificial dermis gets populated with native cells and vascular components. The fibroblasts, replace the bovine collagen to produce the final dermis, resembling regimented normal pattern, rather than the appearance of a scar dermis. After two to three weeks of application, the outer silicone layer is removed and thin skingrafts are applied onto the neo-

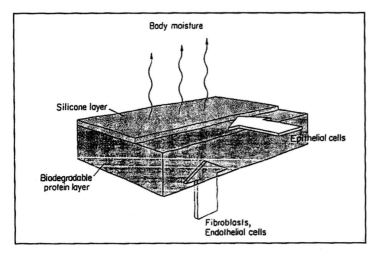

Body moisture

Silicone layer

Epithelial cells

Biodegradable protein layer

Fibroblasts, Endothelial cells

Figure 6.13: Cross-section diagram of bilayered artificial skin, (Integra). Fibroblasts and capillaries migrate into the bottom layer (Collagen and Gag Matrix). While epithelialization proceeds across the surface after removal of the silicone layer and ultra thin split thickness skin grafting (adapted from Jaksic and Burke, Ann Rev med 1987; 38:107-17)

dermis (**Figures 6.14A to C**). No rejection or toxicity has been observed as the artificial dermis gets biodegraded, metabolized and absorbed by the host. The disadvantages are that this material is very expensive and needs at least two surgical procedures for permanent physiological closure of the wound.

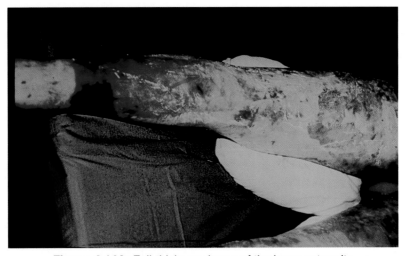

Figure 6.14A: Full-thickness burns of the lower extremity

CULTURED EPIDERMAL AUTOGRAFTS (CEA)

The development of alternative permanent wound closure materials is to incorporate the hosts own cellular and structural components. Tissue culture of epidermal cells obtained from the prospective recipient is of recent technology. Green and Rheinwald described the success of in vitro cultivating and passaging of single suspension of human keratinocytes to produce viable epithelial sheets. Epidermal cells can be cultured into confluent sheets in 21

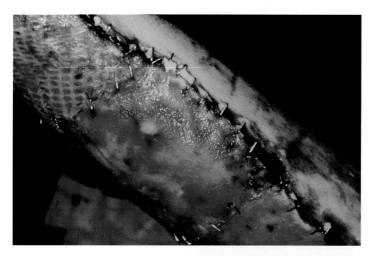

Figure 6.14B: The full-thickness burns after excision and coverage with artificial skin proximaly and meshed autografts distantly on the leg

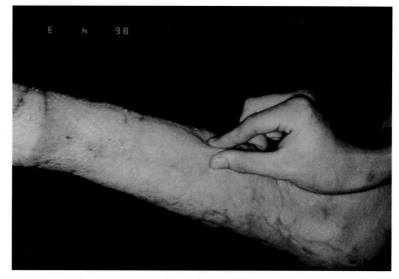

Figure 6.14C: The silicone membrane removed two weeks after application and covered with ultra thin STSG. The picture shows the appearance of the healed wound, 3 months after autografting. The skingraft over integra covered areas is smooth and pliable

days and can be applied to full-thickness burn wounds. Prolonged time of cell culturing is a disadvantage. This time interval is due to failure of many cells to adapt to culture conditions, changes in cell polarity and morphology, shortened lifespan of cells in culture and loss of differentiated characteristics. Extracellular matrix proteins such as fibronectin, laminin, and collagen have a bearing on cell binding. These matrix components either alone or in combination influence cell adhesion, growth, morphology, migration, differentiation, neuronal process and lifespan.

The cultured autografts are used in covering deep burn wounds (Figures 6.15A to C). These cultured epidermal autografts have to be carefully maintained in the wound bed under sterile precautions until they are vascularised and stabilized. The disadvantages are the quality of healing and stability of the healed wound. Since there is no dermal base,

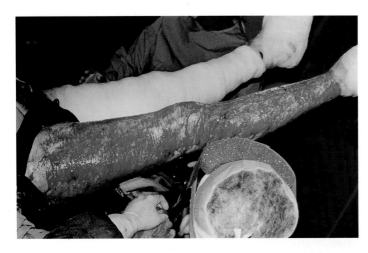

Figure 6.15A: Full thickness burns of the lower extremities; excised to the level of viable tissue

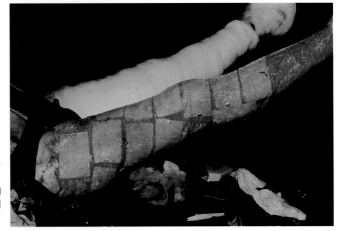

Figure 6.15B: The excised wound being covered with sheets of cultured epidermal autografts

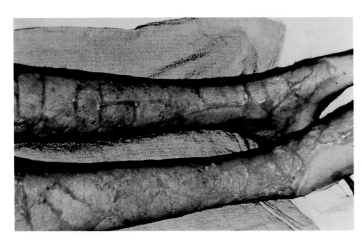

Figure 6.15C: Healed grafts one month after grafting

secondary breakdown of the grafts are common, requiring multiple skingrafting procedures, and scar formation. The culturing procedure is prohibitively expensive and requires two to three weeks of time interval for the permanent closure of the full-thickness burns.

DERMAL SUBSTITUTES

Acellular Dermal Matrix

In recent years, many attempts have been made to produce a dermal substitute capable of supporting skingrafts and cultured epithelial autografts. The most acceptable substitutes produced thus far appears to be those which employ an acellular dermal matrix (ADM) derived from cadaver homograft skin treated to remove epithelial and dermal cellular components. Dermal substitutes must exhibit three important properties: (A) Very low antigenicity. (B) Capacity for rapid vascularization and (C) Stability as a dermal template. None of the ADMS produced by the earlier methods have satisfied these criteria.

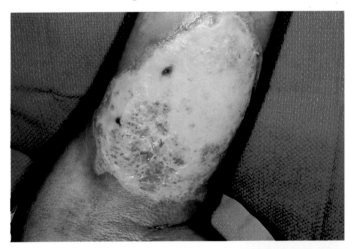

Figure 6.16A: Full-thickness burns on the inner aspect of the arm

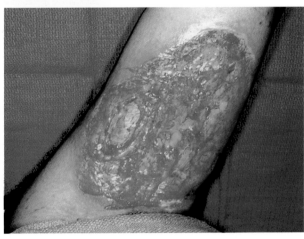

Figure 6.16B: The wound was excised on the 4th post burn day with complete hemostasis

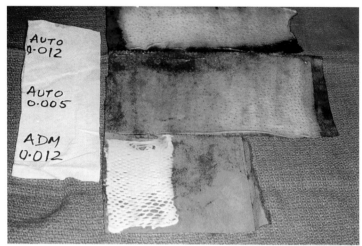

Figure 6.16C: Thick autograft on the top of the picture, thin autograft in the middle and meshed ADM prepared from cadaver homograft at the bottom

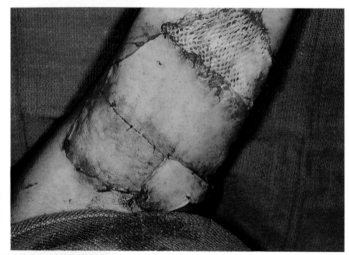

Figure 6.16D: The proximal part of the wound covered with thick sheet grafts and the distal part covered with meshed ADM

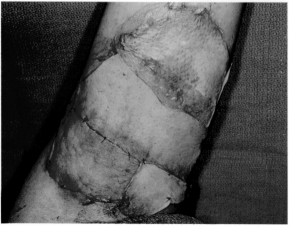

Figure 6.16E: The meshed ADM covered with ultra-thin sheet autograft at the same sitting

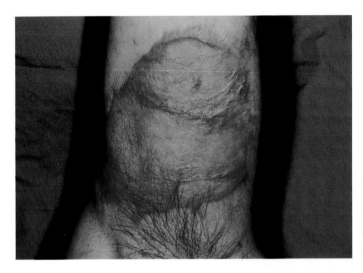

Figure 6.16F: Healed wound three months after grafting. The appearance is same at ADM or thick sheet graft covered areas except at the junction where there was a gap between ADM and thick autograft with scarring

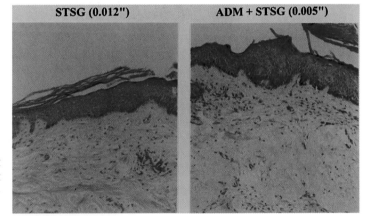

Figure 6.16G: Histological cross-section of the biopsy at thick autograft covered areas and ADM + thin autograft 3 months after grafting. The appearance is essentially same at both areas

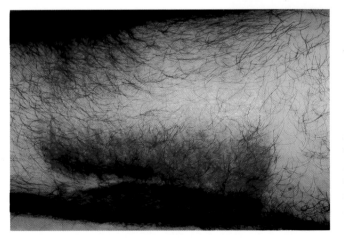

Figure 6.16H: Appearance of the donor site on the thigh three months after harvesting thin (0.005") autografts were taken on the antero-lateral aspects of thigh with minimal discoloration and hypetrophy. Thick (0.012") grafts were harvested on the posterior-lateral aspect of the thigh with persistant discoloration and significant hypertrophy

Recently, more effective and controlled extraction methods using either sodium chloride-sodium didecyl sulfate (Alloderm™) or Dispase-Triton (Walter RJ, Jennings LJ, Matsuda T et al) have been developed. The dermal remnant of the autograft is relatively non-immunogenic, and has served as a recipient layer for thin autograft or cultured keratinocytes. ADM has been used in a one step procedure with a thin overlying autograft **(Figures 6.16A to H)**. It also has been used in combination with cultured keratinocytes. Thinner autografts result in faster donor site healing and therefore, facilitate earlier reharvesting in patients with larger burn injury. Burn surgeons have long recognized that the amount of wound contraction is inversely related to the thickness of the autograft used. Thicker autografts however, increase the risk of unsightly donor site hypertrophy and also visually distracting pigmentation changes. The limitations of ADM are its availability as it is derived from the cadaver homograft.

Dermal Equivalent

Dermal replacement composed of human neonatal fibroblasts cultured on a biodegradable, synthetic matrix (Dermagraft) was developed. Human fibroblasts in contrast to epidermal cells are relatively nonantigenic and thus the constructed dermal tissue replacements could be stored and used readily. Once this dermal replacement is on the wound bed, meshed autograft is applied on it. Vascularisation of the meshed skingraft occurred rapidly in 10 days with subsequent closure of the mesh graft interstices by epithelialisation across the surface of the dermal replacement.

EPIDERMAL-DERMAL COMPOSITE CULTURED GRAFTS

Skin Equivalent

When cultured grafts are placed on full thickness wound, which by definition lacks dermis, there is delayed basement membrane formation with initial development of flat dermal-epidermal junction. This has important consequences on wound healing. Fibroblasts play an important role in the development of basement membrane and associated structures. Bell et.al reported several studies in the early 80's, fabricating living skin equivalent grafts in laboratory with successful application to experimental animals in which they persisted indefinitely. This bilayered skin equivalent composed of sheet of epidermal cells overlying a collagen lattice populated with fibroblasts, quickly became structurally integrated with the surrounding host skin after grafting to Lewis Rats. In 1990, Barbara Hull, a former associate of Dr. Bell, reported successfully treating six patients with a modified skin equivalent. This bilayered skin equivalent consists of an epidermal layer of autologous epidermal cells, and a dermal layer of allogenic fibroblasts with collagen.

These skin equivalents, when applied and taken successfully, provide epidermis and dermis in one stage. They greatly minimize donor site extent, depth; provide permanent and life-saving wound closure.

These skin equivalents require further refinements in fabrication and application. They are not available for general clinical use at this time.

BIBLIOGRAPHY

1. Atnip, Robert G, Burke, John F: Skin Coverage. *Current problems in surgery* **10**: 1983.
2. Baxter CR: Homograft and heterografts as a biologic dressing in the treatment of thermal injury. Presented at the First Annual Congress of the Society of German Plastic Surgeons, Munich, September 9, 1970.
3. Bell E, Ehrlich HP, Sher S *et al*: Development and use of a living skin equivalent. *Plast Reconstr Surg* **67**: 386-92, 1981.
4. Bose B: "Burn wound dressing with human amniotic membrane. *Annals R Coll Surg Eng* **61**: 444, 1979
5. Browne, Earl Z Jr: Skingrafts in operative hand surgery.
6. Burke JF, Yannas IV, Quinby WC *et al*: Successful use of a physiologically acceptable artificial skin in the treatment of extensive burn injury. *Ann Surg* **194**:413-28, 1981.
7. Burleson R, Eiseman B: Mechanisms of antibacterial effect of biological dressings. *Ann Surg* **171**: 181-186,1973.
8. Gallico GG, O' Connor NE, Compton CC *et al*: Permanent coverage of large burn wounds with autologous cultured human epithelium. *N Engl J Med* **311**: 448-451, 1984.
9. Gary F, Purdue John L, Hunt, Robert W *et al*: "Biosynthetic skin substitute versus frozen human cadaver allograft for temporary coverage of excised burn wounds. *Jour of Trauma* **27**:2, 1987.
10. Haberal M, Oner Z, Bayraktar V *et al*: The use of silver sulfadiazine incorporated amniotic membrane as a temporary dressing. *Burns* **13**: 159, 1987.
11. Hansbrough *et al*: Clinical experience with biobrane synthetic dressing in the treatment of partial-thickness burns. *Burns* **10**:415, 1984.
12. Hansbrough JF: Wound coverage with biologic dressings and cultured skin substitutes. RG Landes, Co., 1992.
13. Herndon DH: Total burn care, WB Saunders Co. Ltd. **1**: 1996.
14. Hickerson, W and Compton C: The use of cultured epidermal autografts over dermal allografts to close major burn wounds. *Proc 23rd Amer Burn Assoc*, **7**:1991.
15. Hickerson W, Compton C, Fetchall S *et al*: Cultured epidermal autografts and allodermis combination for permanent burn wound coverage. *Burns* **20 (1)**: S52-56, 1994.
16. Kealey GP *et al*: Cadaver skin allografts and transmission of human cytomegalovirus to burn patients. *J Am Coll Surg* **182**:201-205, 1996.
17. May SR *et al*: Recent Developments in skin banking and the clinical uses of cryopreserved skin. *J Med Assoc Georgia* 233-236, 1984.
18. Pensler JM, Mulliken JB: Skingrafts: To mesh or not to mesh. *Contemporary Surgery* **32**: 45,1988.
19. Pigeon J. Treatment of second degree burns with amniotic membranes. *Can Med Assoc J* **83**: 844 1960.
20. Piserchia NE, Akenzua GI: Amniotic membrane dressings in burns in children. A cheap method of treatment for developing countries. *Trop Geor Med* **33**: 235, 1981.
21. Pruitt BA, Levine NS. Characteristics and uses of biological dressings and skin substitutes. *Arch Surg* **19**:312,1984.
22. Pruitt BA Jr, Silverstein P: Methods of resurfacing denuded skin areas. *Transpl Proc* **3**: 1537-1545, 1971.
23. Pruitt BA, Levine NS: Characteristics and uses of biologic dressings and skin substitutes. *Arch Surg* **119**:312-322,1984.
24. Purna Sai K, Mary Babu. Collagen based dressings: A review. *Burns* **26**: 54-62, 2000.
25. Ramakrishnan KM, Doss CR, Rao DK: Human amniotic membrane as a temporary biological dressing in complicated burns in a developing country. *J Burn Care Rehabil* **4**: 202-204, 1983.
26. Ramakrishnan KM, Jayaraman V: Management of partial thickness wounds by amniotic membrane — a cost effective treatment in developing countries. *Burns* **23**:s33-s36, 1997.
27. Robson *et al*: Synthetic skin dressings: Round table discussion. *JBCR* **6**:66, 1985.
28. Robson MC, Krizek TJ: Clinical experiences with amniotic membrane as a temporary biologic dressing. *CaaMed* **38**: 449, 1974.
29. Robson Martin C: Predicting skingraft survival. *J Trauma* **13**: 213,1973.

30. Salisbury R, Wilmore D, Silverstein P: Biological dressings for skingraft donor sites. *Arch Surg* **106:** 7105-706, 1973.

31. Sawhney CP: Amniotic membrane as a biological dressing in the management of burns. *Burns* **15:** 339-342, 1989

32. Shuck JM, Pruitt BA, Moncrief JA: Homograft skin for wound coverage. *Arch Surg* **98:** 472-479, 1969.

33. Srivatsava A., Desagun E, Jennings *et al*: Use of procine acellular dermal matrix as a dermal substitute in rats. *Annals of Surgery* **233**:3, 2001.

34. Teepe RGC, Kreis RW, Koebrugge EJ *et al*: The use of cultured autologous epidermis in the treatment of extensive burn wounds. *J Trauma* **30:** 269-275, 1990.

35. Turner TD. Semiocclusive and occlusive dressing. An environment for healing. The role of occlusion. London UK. Royal Society of Medicine International congress and symposium, **67:** 93-107,1985.

36. Viswanatha Rao T, Chandrasekaran V: Use of dry human and bovine amnion as a biological dressing. *Arch Surg* **117:** 116, 1981.

37. Wainwright D, Madden M, Luterman A *et al*: Clinical evaluation an acellular allograft dermal matrix in full-thickness burns. *J Burn Care Rehabil* **17:** 124-136, 1996.

38. Waler RJ, Matsuda T, Reyes H *et al*: Charecterization of acellular dermal matrices (ADMS) prepared by two different methods. *Burns* **24**:2, 1998.

39. Walter RJ, Jennings LJ, Matsuda T *et al*: Dispase/Triton treated acellular dermal matrix as a dermal substitute in rats. *Current Surgery* **54:** 6, 1997.

40. Winter GD: Formation of the scar and the rate of epithelialisation of superficial wounds in the skin of the young domestic pig. *Nature* **193:** 293-4, 1962.

7

Pharmacological Modulation of the Burn Wound

INTRODUCTION

The anatomic discontinuity of the skin caused by physical, chemical, or thermal insult is restored by a mechanism of wound repair. Wound healing is an orderly, integrated, dynamic process comprised of multiple temporally and spatially overlapping but distinct phases, namely inflammation, vascularization, fibroplasia, reepithelializaion, and remodeling. The biological signals released during the initial clot formation and throughout the repair modulate controlled migration, proliferation and differentiation of cells actively involved in this event leading to wound closure. This process is completed by the synthesis of extracellular matrix proteins in appropriate quantity and quality. Considerable advances made in understanding cell-cell and cell-matrix interactions in cutaneous wound healing provide evidence for a critical role of matrix in influencing cell migration, polarity, and orientation. The formation of surface epithelium to close the wound is precisely orchestrated with the underlying dermal repair. This synchrony is key to preventing either insufficient or excess wound repair.

Chronic wounds are a major world health problem resulting in distress and disability on the elderly and an increasing burden to health care providers. Chronic wounds exist in the following forms - pressure sores, venous ulcers and diabetic ulcers. In normal wound healing the repair of the epithelial and mesenchymal tissues of the skin is effected by keratinocytes, endothelial cells and fibroblast and coordinated via complex cell/cell and cell/matrix interactions. These responses are altered in chronic wounds with prolonged inflammation, a defective wound matrix and failure of reepithelialisation. Wound surface supports a diverse microspores and these microorganisms contribute to non-healing.

INFLAMMATORY PHASE

Burn injury is followed by various biological and metabolic alterations which include changes in activity of certain serum proteins, enzymes and significant reduction in polyunsaturated fatty acids in the red cell membrane. The rate of healing may depend on metabolic conditions as well as response elicited in the tissue site due to injury. The major enzymatic changes take place during the first phase of healing, the inflammatory phase, and it plays a key role, as it is the decisive phase of wound healing. The reaction of vascularized tissue to local injury is defined as inflammation. The characteristic feature of inflammatory process in higher forms is the reaction of blood vessels, leading to the accumulation of fluids and blood cells.

Inflammation serves to destroy, dilute or wall-off the injurious agents, but in turn it sets into motion a series of events that heal and reconstitute the damaged tissue. The inflammatory response is closely intertwined with the process of repair. The repair begins during the early phase of inflammation but reaches completion usually after the injurious influence has been neutralized. The causative factors of the inflammation include microbial infection, physical agents (such as radiation and trauma), chemicals (toxins and caustic substances), necrotic tissue and all type of immunological reactions. The processes of inflammation are classified as acute and chronic. During acute inflammation exudation of fluid, plasma proteins (acute phase proteins) and the emigration of leukocytes (predominantly neutrophils) occur. It is also noticed that the acute phase response due to burn injury persists longer than is observed with other trauma (surgery, infection etc.,). This has been accounted for by the metabolic depression early after injury, to increased catabolism and elimination of certain proteins from the vascular space and may also be due to differences in rates of synthesis. Chronic inflammation is characterized by the presence of lymphocytes and macrophage in the injured and regenerating tissue with proliferation of blood vessels and connective tissue. Many of the vascular and cellular response of the inflammation are mediated by chemical factors derived from the action of the inflammatory stimulus on plasma or cells. However overwhelming inflammation due to excess stimulation of these chemicals may have deleterious effects on wound healing.

ACUTE PHASE RESPONSE

The inflammation is accompanied by a large number of systemic and metabolic changes, which are referred to collectively as the acute phase response. The acute phase response is characterized by a set of hepatic disturbances which include marked variations in the concentration of some plasma proteins. Those proteins whose concentrations increase are referred to as positive acute phase proteins, those whose levels decline are termed negative acute phase proteins. These changes occur in a uniform, predictable manner and are a common response to nearly all forms of injury regardless of the excitatory agent. Acute phase proteins pattern varies form one species to another. Thus, C-reactive proteins and serum amyloid A show the highest increase in man, whereas in rats, α_2-macroglobulin and α_1-acid glycoprotein exhibit the most substantial increases. In many species, plasma concentrations of fibrinogen, α_1-antitrypsin, haptoglobin and α_1-antichymotrypsin increase and, simultaneously, albumin and transferrin plasma levels decrease. Evaluation of these plasma proteins change are of considerable significance in determining the effectiveness of certain antiinflammatory drugs in animals.

First phase of healing is composed mainly of fibronectin and fibrin. Later on plasmin, the body's own fibrinolytic agent, breaks down the fibrin barrier to restore circulation. As a response to trauma the liver releases acute-phase proteins such as α_1-antitrypsin and (α_2-macroglobulin which bind to plasmin and hence fibrinolysis is shut down. C-reactive protein, another acute-phase protein, serves as an indicator of the status of the inflammatory process. Here the study has been made to understand the physiological factors responsible for inflammation and consequent edema formation, and the beneficial effects of trypsin:chymotrypsin

(Chymoral Forte DS-Elder Pharmaceuticals, India) by analysing qualitatively and quantitatively changes in serum acute phase proteins. Chymoral Forte is approved by drug controller in India for administration in surgical conditions to reduce inflammation. This enzyme prepration was trypsin: chymotrypsin in the ratio of 6 : 1 with an enzymatic activity of 200,00 AU/tablet. Four tablets per day were administered orally from day 1 of admission and then daily for 10 days for the treated group of patients. Thirty patients with 20 to 30 percent deep second degree burn (20-50 years) with severe clinical edema were investigated. The patients were grouped into two categories. Group I (n = 15) were not treated with chymoral forte and served as control; Group II (n = 15) patients were treated with trypsin: Chymotrypsin preparation. Blood samples were collected from day 1 of admission and then daily for 10 days from both the groups of patients. Immediately after collection, blood samples were centrifuged and serum was separated and stored at -20°C until use. Hence, the study was carried out with trypsin:chymotrypsin combination to see if the action of acute-phase proteins on fibrinolytic shut down can be minimized and the severity of the inflammatory phase could be reduced. To study the effect of these preparation three acute-phase proteins, namely C-reactive protein, α_1-antitrypsin and α_2-macroglobulin were taken into consideration. The greater homology between α_1-antitrypsin and α_1-antichymotrypsin led to the selection of α_1-antitrypsin for a detailed study.

Unlike the change in some other acute-phase reaction, the rise in C-reactive protein correlates well with the extent of injury or tissue destruction. It has been suggested that there is a close correlation between the level of C-reactive protein to the area, depth and severity of a burn, the lower post-burn titer values of C-reactive protein in the enzyme treated group than the control group in our study suggest that the enzyme has acted effectively during the initial phase and reduced the degree of inflammation, and that probably resulted in the reduction of C-reactive protein titer value in treated groups (**Figure 7.1**).

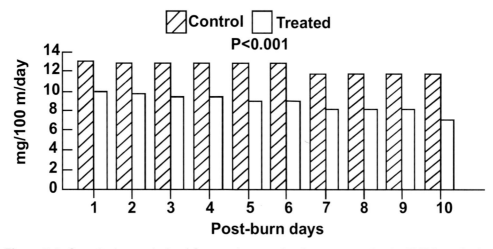

Figure 7.1: Quantitative analysis of C - reactive protein of serum samples by ELISA method

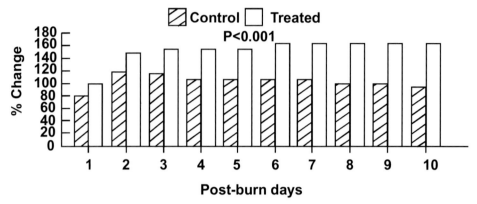

Figure 7.2: Trypsin inhibitory capacity of serum samples

The protective actions of acute-phase reactants are that they inactivate the damaging proteases like neutrophil elastase and cathepsin G. The higher titer values of α_1-antitrypsin in the enzyme-treated groups than the controls observed in this study clearly indicated that the difference is enzyme dependent. Such high titer values helped to minimize the activity of neutral proteases (elastase, cathepsin G etc.,) released from disrupted polymorphonuclear leucocytes at the site of inflammation. As is seen from these studies there is an increase in titer values of α_1-antitrysin in the enzyme treated groups, hence there should be a comparable rise in the functional capacity of the serum to inhibit trypsin. The reported trypsin inhibitory capacity (TIC) of the serum confirms the correlation between the increased titer values of TIC and α_1-antitrypsin in enzyme treated groups (**Figures 7.2 and 7.3**). A possible physiological role of α_2-macroglobulin in the treated group signifies that the changes had occurred only due to the oral enzyme administration, in contrast to the very limited changes generally seen following trauma alone.

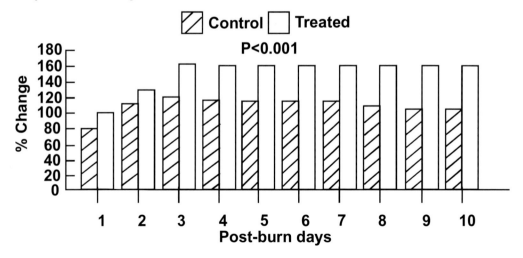

Figure 7.3: Quantitative analysis of α_1-Antitrypsin of serum samples

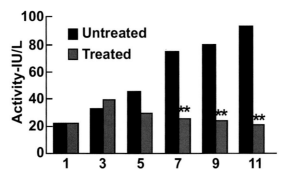

Figure 7.4: Changes in the activity of serum glutamate pyruvate transaminase

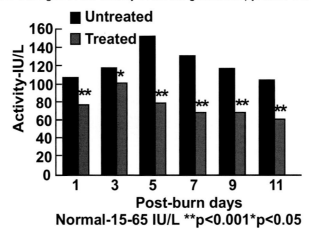

Normal-15-65 IU/L **p<0.001*p<0.05

Figure 7.5: Changes in the activity of serum alkaline phosphatase

SERUM MARKER ENZYMES

The inflammatory changes that occur in the system may alter the levels of enzymes, which serve as an indicator for various diseases. In this condition the measurement of certain marker serum (SGPT, SGOT, CPK, ALP, LDH) and proteolytic (cathepsin D and elastase) enzymes may be helpful. Previous studies show that burn size (TBSA), inhalation injury, severe shock and systemic infection are closely related to the occurrence of multiple organ failure. The measurement of SGPT, SGOT, CPK, ALP, LDH on post-burn days 1-10 will serve as a useful criterion in assessing the possibility of myocardial infarction,: haemolysis, acute liver and muscle damage. The proteolytic enzyme release during the phagocytosis may prolong inflammation and increase tissue damage. For this reason the administration of anti-inflammatory drugs are used to limit the normal inflammatory reaction. The ideal drug would be one that enhances the salutary effects of inflammation, yet controls its harmful sequelae. The present study clearly demonstrated that the enzyme preparation (trypsin: chymotrypsin) appears to have a protective role in decreasing the activities of serum enzymes levels in the treated group when compared with untreated, suggesting that there is a limitation of the damage to various organs like heart, muscle and other tissues **(Figures 7.4 to 7.7)**. The

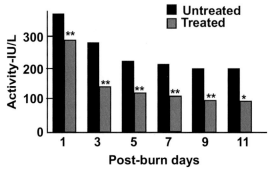

Figure 7.6: Changes in the activity of serum creatine phosphokinase

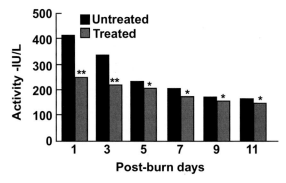

Figure 7.7: Changes in the activity of serum lactate dehydrogenase

Table 7.1: Proteolytic enzymes (Cathepsin D and elastase) activities during post-burn periods

	Post-burn days					
	1	3	5	7	9	11
Cathepsin Dn = 9.83+0.463						
Burns untreated	19.15±0.200	16.01±0.060	14.96±0.115	13.29+0.080	12.2210.064	11.12±0.075
Burns treated	15.27***±0.195	13.18**±0.087	11.10**±0.070.	11.01**±0.109	10.89**±0.031	10.0r*±0.038
Elastase n = 0.245 ± 0.007						
Burns untreated	0.635 ±0.007	0.556±0.002	0.445 ±0.002	0.421 ±0.004	0.359 ±0.003	0.355 ±0.001
Burns treated	0.554***±0.002	0.440'*±0.001	0.372**±0.003	0.322**±0.002	0.301**±0.002	0.265**±0.001

Untreated Vs treated: ***P<0.001; **P<0.01.
All values are mean±SEM of six samples.

trypsin:chymotrypsin combination used in our study to treat burn patients served as a good anti-inflammatory agent by reducing the burn edema and enhancing the process of healing. As already shown in our earlier studies, there was an increase in the levels of acute phase proteins (α_1-antitrypsin and α_2-macroglobulin) in cases of treated patients. The high levels account for the decrease in the activities of cathepsin D and elastase in the treated groups, as α_1-antitrypsin and α_2-macroglobulin may bind to the proteases and thus cause inactivation (Table 7.1). This becomes an important clearance mechanism for removal of proteolytic enzyme from the circulation.

OXIDATIVE DAMAGE AND ANTIOXIDANTS

It has been well documented that after trauma or burn injury a cytokine cascade is activated, with subsequent stimulation of phagocytic cells that result in the formation of oxygen free radicals leading to lipid peroxidation. Polymorphonuclear cell degranulation has been considered as a primary source of oxygen free radical after burn injury. Oxidation of polyunsaturated fatty acids from membrane phospholipids may produce additional free radicals, which in turn stimulate further lipid peroxidation and tissue injury. This lipid peroxidation process appears to continue as long as the inflammation persists. The generation of free radicals in the absence of scavenging defenses might be the major cause of some acute and chronic disease. But the natural scavengers of free radicals may come to the rescue and offer protection against cellular damage. Effective natural scavengers of free radicals consist of a number of enzymatic and non-enzymatic antioxidants. Enzymatic antioxidants include superoxide dismutase (SOD), catalase, glutathione peroxidase (GPX) and glutathione s-transferase (GST). Nonenzymatic antioxidants are lipid soluble α-tocopherol and water soluble ascorbic acid apart from ceruloplasmin and haptoglobin. The enzymatic antioxidants carry specific metal ions (at the active site) as prosthetic group, which comes under the classification of trace elements.

It is well-known that burn injury necessitates increased nutritional requirements associated with the resulting hypermetabolic state. Among the nutrients required for supplementation, trace elements need greater attention because stress alters the level of these trace elements due to altered intestinal absorption, altered body losses, altered distribution among body proteins and altered protein concentrations. Different trace elements have specific roles to play during the process of healing. Copper is an essential nutrient and has several functions as an integral component of numerous enzymes. One such enzyme is ceruloplasmin, which has ferroxidase activity. Small amounts of selenium are needed for tissue oxygenation and for protection against lipid peroxidation. Iron is important in energy metabolism because of its structural role in oxygen carrying proteins. It is also associated with various enzymes including catalase, GPX and various dehydrogenases. Zinc, a trace element plays most important role in wound healing in addition to its role in RNA and protein synthesis. Inhibitors of oxygen radicals generating systems such as allopurinol, physiologic enzyme scavengers, i.e., SOD and catalase, physiologic antioxidants such as tocopherol or glutathione have been used in experimentally induced shock.

The results observed in our present study on the administration of trypsin:chymotrypsin preparation in burn patients clearly indicate a reduction in lipid peroxidation products (**Figure 7.8**). In the present study we attribute the higher levels of SOD, catalase, glutathione peroxidase, gluatathione-s-transferase, and ceruloplasmins maintained for a longer period of time during treatment to the effective scavenging of the oxygen free radicals (**Figures 7.8 to 7.10**).

The enzyme preparation (trypsin:chymotrypsin) apart from playing the role as an anti-inflammatory agent has also been proved to serve indirectly as an effective antioxidant by reducing the tissue destruction and decreasing the free radical formation and thereby maintaining the antioxidant levels for a longer period of time.

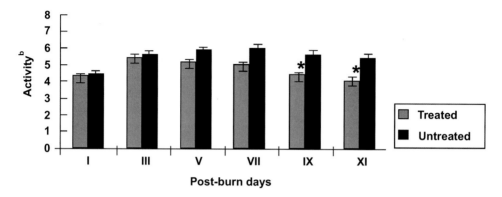

Figure 7.8: Changes in the lipid peroxidation product (malondialdehyde) levels in treated and untreated groups

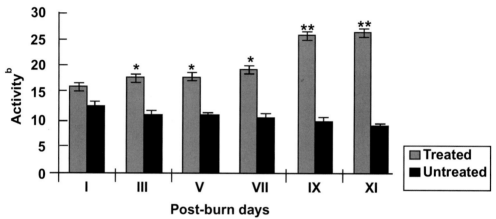

Figure 7.9: Catalase levels in treated and untreated groups

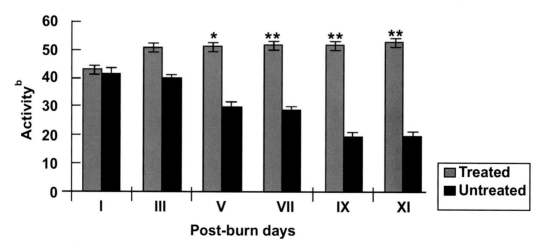

Figure 7.10: Superoxide dismutase levels in treated and untreated groups

Nitric oxide (NO) plays an important role in many physiological and pathological processes. It is produced in different mammalian cells by nitric oxide synthase which converts L- arginine to L- citrulline. There are 2 important isoforms, a constitutive enzyme c-nitric oxide synthetase and an inducible enzyme i- nitric oxide synthase which produce large amount of nitric oxide. The excess production of nitric oxide can cause the oxidative damage of tissue by forming peroxynitrite with superoxide anion. Peroxynitrite is a potent oxidant, it reacts with many cellular lipids and protein components thereby disturbing their function. It was shown that administration of a specific inhibitor of i-nitric oxide synthase, namely s-methyl isothiourea (SMT) after thermal injury suppressed i-nitric oxide synthase activity. This resulted in the decreased formation of peroxynitrite and subsequently reduced the oxidative damage in tissues.

Specific inhibition of i-nitric oxide synthase decreases the interstitial mucosal peroxynitrite level and improves the barrier function after thermal injury. The protective effect of SOD compounds, copper-zinc SOD and manganese SOD was investigated in burn injury and proved to be effective in preventing tissue damage.

Highly reactive free radicals released from neutrophil lead to the generation of lipid peroxides. Sulfhydryl containing compounds especially reduced glutathione (GSH) are important in the protection of cells against hydroperoxide damage. The effects of N-acetyl cysteine (NAC) an antioxidant was investigated. This compound besides being a scavenger of hydroxyl radical was found to increase GSH levels after burn injury, thus minimizing lipid peroxidation in tissues. Hence the addition of NAC to the protocols for the treatment of burn patients is suggested.

The effect of antioxidant therapy on cell mediated immunity following burn injury was investigated in an animal model. To prevent lipid peroxidation and free radical formation or to scavenge toxic oxygen metabolites ibuprofen, allopurinol, catalase, superoxide dismutase, desferroxamine, glutathione, N- acetyl cysteine (NAS), vitamin C, vitamin E have been used to improve post-burn tissue injury and organ dysfunction. Ibuprofen restored immunity after burn injury by blocking prostaglandin synthesis and it is also known to decrease oxygen radical release from neutrophils, its protective effect was studied in burn experimental models.

PROINFLAMMATORY CYTOKINES

Cytokines are produced during the effector phases of natural and specific immunity and serve to mediate, and regulate immuno, and inflammatory responses. The cytokines that mediate natural immunity include those, which protect against viral infection and those that initiate inflammatory reactions to protect against bacteria. Among the cytokines, interleukin-6 (IL-6) is a pleotrophic cytokine with multiple effects on many systems. Induction of acute phase reactants in hepatic cells, B-cell differentiation, and proliferation, and differentiation of T-cells are observed with IL-6. The production of IL-6 in these cells is regulated, either positively or negatively by a variety of signals including mitogens, antigenic stipulations, IL-1β, PDGF and viruses. The various activities of IL-β and IL-6 suggest that they have a major role in the mediation of inflammatory and immune responses initiated by infection or injury.

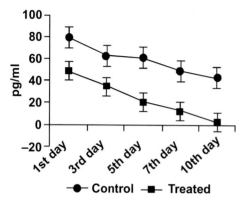

Figure 7.11A: Serum IL-6 Levels in burn patients (16 - 20% TBSA)

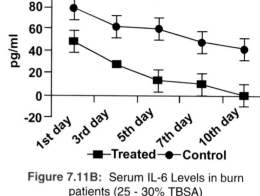

Figure 7.11B: Serum IL-6 Levels in burn patients (25 - 30% TBSA)

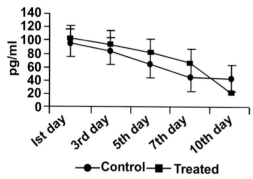

Figure 7.11C: Serum IL-6 Levels in burn patients (25 - 34% Sepsis)

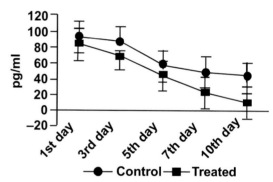

Figure 7.11D: Serum IL-6 Levels in burn patients (35 - 40% TBSA)

Results obtained by us also showed that there was a good response to cytokines by drug treatment and levels of serum IL-lβ and IL-6 declined within about 4 to 5 days post-burn. Circulating IL-lβ and IL-6 levels of trypsin-chymotrypsin preparation treated cases remained relatively low after 6-10 days of the treatment. Our investigation clearly established the modulation of proinflammatory cytokines IL-lβ and IL-6 by trypsin-chymotrypsin preparations and it is worthwhile looking at the expression of anti-inflammatory cytokines during drug treatment to understand in depth the pathophysiology of burn injury (Figures 7.11A to D).

All these acquired data demonstrate the effect of oral enzyme administration to burn patients on certain early phases of inflammation. The enzyme helps in minimizing the initial chronic acute inflammatory response and helps in free plasmin availability for fibrinolytic action, subsequently resulting in suppression of edema. This oral enzyme proves to be advantageous as it moderates a normal physiological mechanism during the initial phase of healing and helps in the reduction of necrotic stage thereby quickening the process of healing.

HEPARIN THERAPY

We have also investigated the efficacy of heparin treatment in burn wound healing. Heparin, a highly sulfated glycosoaminoglycan studied originally for its anticoagulant property has been dealt in a new prospective as an anti-inflammatory agent. Nevertheless that heparin facilitates wound healing and shortens the recovery period in thermal burns was established already in Guinea pigs and in clinical trials in burn patients.

Heparin is postulated to play a positive role in angiogenesis or neovascularization and this process of formation of new blood vessels is an important step in wound healing. Heparin is proposed to be an anti-inflammatory agent and we are interested in assessing this property of heparin with respect to modulation of IL-6 levels during inflammatory phase of healing.

Thirty patients with 25 to 35 % TBSA superficial partial thickness, and deep partial thickness by flame, chemical and electrical burns were selected for the study with prior permission. Among 30 patients, 15 patients were treated with Heparin, 100,000 IU stat followed by 10,000 IU subcutaneous under PTT control daily for 6 to 10 days and the remaining patients served as controls. The first blood sample was collected at the time of admission to the burn center and subsequent samples on days 3, 5, 7, 10, and 12. IL-6 levels in serum were determined. The degree and type of inflammatory cell infiltration during the process of healing and collagen deposition was monitored in the punch biopsy samples.

The following parameters were assessed for the clinical observations of heparin treated patients and control:

1. Regression of oedema
2. Absence of erythema
3. Eschar formation
4. Arrest of progressive necrosis
5. Rate of epithelialisation
   Serum IL-6 levels decreased in heparin treated patients much earlier than the control patients. Beneficial clinical effects have been endorsed with the measurement of serum IL-6
6. The earlier wound healing in heparin treated group of deep partial thickness burn wounds was due to the reduction in IL-6 levels by heparin administration (Figure 7.12).

Tissue Remodeling in Heparin Therapy

The biopsy samples collected in the wound area on Day 5,10,15,20 and 25 post-burn were processed for histochemical analysis.

On the 5th day, in the treated cases cellular infiltration is reduced whereas untreated cases show increased inflammatory cells and the early necrosis of the epidermis as a result of burn is obvious. Collagen deposited in the dermis is being organised in the treated cases on the 10th day, whereas it looks haphazard in the control cases.

By day 15, dermal collagen organization parallel to the epithelial surface correlates well with epidermal regeneration and differentiation in the treated patients, but the controls still lack dermal organisation and epidermal regeneration.

Evidence of complete remodeled skin is obvious on the 25th day in treated cases whereas

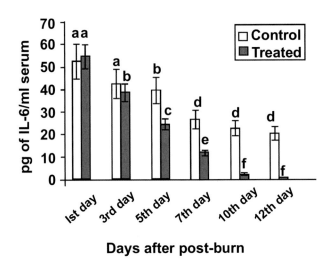

Figure 7.12: Changes of serum IL-6 levels in heparin treated and control burn patients [25% TBSA, Figure 7.1]. Immunosorbent ELISA linked serum interleukine -6 levels in heparin treated and control burn patients, n = 6, (DMRT one way ANOVA) similar letters in bar represents no significant differences at $p < 0.05$ level

epithelial debris on the wound surface is still seen in the control cases and the dermal region also is not completely matured and organised. Thus, accelerated wound healing in heparin treatment is attributed to controlled inflammatory phase in burn patients.

The anticoagulant heparin sodium conventional therapy produced significant favorable alteration in experimental thermal burns in dogs, rabbits, and rats. The beneficial effects were evident in thermal burns of humans when Saliba and Griner used large dose of heparin administered both parenterally and topically.

Heparin has been widely used under controlled conditions in extensive burns systemically to prevent intravascular coagulation producing shock lung syndrome and locally by way of aerosol preparation of dressings. In humans, heparin consistently relieved pain due to burns and balanced erythema. Importantly, the inflammation in the burn area increases the swelling or edema and in heparin treated burn patients swelling has been subsidized and did not reappear. Heparin treated burns in humans and Guinea pigs became progressively reduced in size and were comparatively smaller in heparin treated pigs than the control and significant reduction in burn wound size was observed within 9 to 11 days.

Several heparin-binding growth factors (HBGFs) are thought to play a key role in natural processes of tissue regeneration after release from inflammatory or circulating cells. It was postulated that, heparin like bipolymers constitute a new family of tissue repair agents with wide variety of potential use in wound management strategies and it could be explored in impaired healing associated with diabetes.

Heparin influences the regulation of angiogenesis and it has a chemotactic effect on endothelial cells in human cell cultures and potentiate the chemotactic activity of endothelial cell growth factor (ECGF), with resultant stimulation of neovascularization. These effects on

Heparin treated

Control

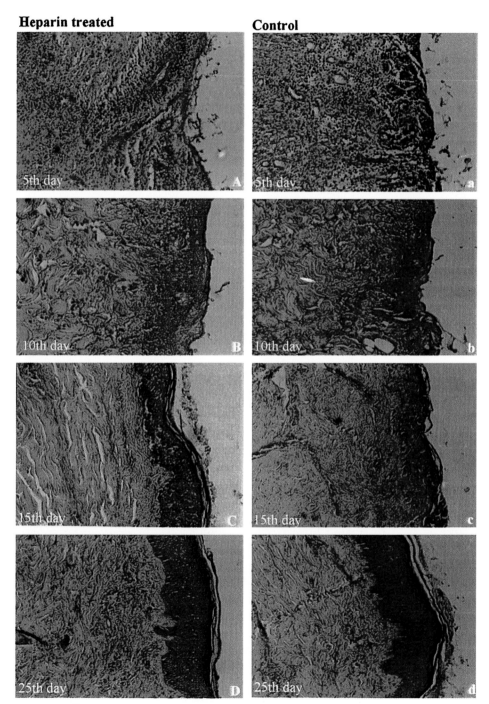

Figure 7.13: Tissue remodeling in heparin treated and control burn
patients visualised by H and E staining

endothelial cell migration and angiogenesis may be relevant to reported observation of improved wound healing after heparin treatment.

Our present study showed that heparin treatment was effective in reducing burn edema and reduction in IL-6, the proinflammatory cytokine activity and also hastened wound epithelialisation and thus burn wound healing was early and scar outcome is good. Control cases showed delayed regression of burn edema, decreased rate of epithelialisation, and the cytokine expression showed significant variation from heparin treated patients. The earlier wound healing in heparin treated group of partial thickness burn wounds was due to the reduction in IL-6 levels by heparin treatment **(Figures 7.12 and 7.13)**.

CONCLUSION

One of the authors in the group of investigators observed the above beneficial effects of using Trypsin: Chymotrypsin and Heparin in burn patients, which modified the inflammatory phase resulting in accelerated would healing. These studies are still in progress with more number of patients in different degrees of burn injury.

(The investigations of Chymoral Forte DS therapy in Burn patients described in the chapter "Pharmacological Modulation of the Burn Wound" has been published in the BURNS journal, Elsevier Science Ltd., and the references cited. The permission granted by the Editor of BURNS, Dr. Peter G. Shakespere to include the study in this chapter is gratefully acknowledged).

BIBLIOGRAPHY

1. Davies JWL: *Physiological Responses to Burning Injury,* London, Academic Press, 425,1982.
2. Glenn EM, Bowman BJ, Koslowske TC: *Chemical Biology of Inflammation,* New York, Pergamon Press, 1968.
3. Kushner L: The phenomenon of the acute phase response *Ann NY Acad Sci* 389, 39-48, 1982.
4. Latha B, Mathangi Ramakrishnan, JayaramanV, Mary Babu: The efficacy of trypsin: chymotrypsin preparation in the reduction of oxidative damage during burn injury, *Burns,* 24, 532-538, 1998.
5. Latha B, Mathangi Ramakrishnan, Jayaraman V, Mary Babu: Serum enzymatic changes modulated using trypsin: Chymotrypsin preparation during burn wounds in humans, *Burns,* 23, 560-564, 1997.
6. Latha B, Ramakrishnan KM, Jayaraman V: Action of trypsin: Chymotrypsin (Chymoral forte DS) preparation on acute-phase proteins following burn injury in humans, *Burns,* 23, S3-S7, 1997.
7. Mary Babu, Alan Wells: Dermal-epidermal communication in wound healing, *Wounds,*13,183-189, 2001.
8. Ramakrishnan KM, Babu M, Ramachandran K: "Altered Pattern of Collagen Synthesis in Burns treated with Systemic and local heparin". In VIIIth Congress of IPRS transactions, Montreal, Canada, 1984.
9. Ravikumar T, Mathangi Ramakrishnan, Jayaraman V, Mary Babu: Effect of trypsin-chymotrypsin (Chymoral forte DS) preparation on the modulation of cytokine levels in burns patients, *Burns,* 27, 709-716, 2001.
10. Ryan G, Majno G: Acute inflammation, a review. *American Journal of Pathology,* 86, 185, 1977.
11. Saliba MJ Jr: Heparin in the treatment of burns: a review. *Burns,* 27, 349-358, 2001.
12. Saliba MJ Jr: The effects and the use of heparin in the care of burns that improves treatment and enhances the quality of life. *Acta Chirur Plast* 39,13-16, 1997.
13. Wilhelm DL: Inflammation and healing. In: *Pathology* Anderson WAD (Ed), 6th edition, CV Mosby, 1(6):4-67, 1971.

8

Early Surgical Management of the Burn Wound

Traditional management of burn wound in the past, consisted of daily wound cleansing with blunt and sharp debridement of minimally adherent necrotic tissue. The eschar separated because of the action of collagenase from bacteria and the debridements. Granulation tissue formed in the base of the wound, and ultimately skin grafting of the wound was accomplished. The skin grafts would become viable if the bacterial count in the wound was low enough and shearing forces were controlled. Vigorous occupational and physical therapy was then undertaken to maximize movement, strength and all of this was accomplished with great pain. The present state of burn care includes early surgical excision and closure of the burn wound. Excision of burns was originally accomplished in 1891 by Lustgarten. Dr. Oliver Cope cared for patients in the 1942 coconut grove fire and noted that patients with excision did better than others. The invention of the dermatome and the skin mesher were great advances in wound closure that allowed excisional therapy to be an option. Advances in blood banking, anesthesia, and critical care have allowed us to perform previously unthinkable procedures, including burn excisions.

At present, most burn centers in the USA utilize surgical excisional therapy of the burn wound. When surgical excision and subsequent wound closure is obtained in selected cases, infection and sepsis are diminished, nutritional requirements are diminished, hospital stay is decreased, and pain of the wound is decreased.

Surgical excision and wound closure may produce less severe contractures, and better *aesthetic* result.

Removal of necrotic tissue is a surgical principle which certainly makes sound physiological sense. To leave dead tissue on the patient until bacterial proliferation separates the necrotic tissue leaves the patient at great risk of infection and its detrimental effects. With the development of the Burn Team concept, the ability to remove the dead tissue and replace it with similar tissue, i.e. skin grafts, is possible now a days in most cases.

The problem of an adequate amount of skin replacement for the massively burned patient remains a major concern. However much creative work is being done and hopefully, the problem will be conquered in the next few years. Temporary and permanent wound closure techniques were discussed in the previous chapter. Certainly surgical excision of the burn wound should not be accomplished unless the wound can be closed at the same time.

The patient population to be offered burn excisional therapy depends upon the depth of the wound, the etiology of the injury, the location of the burn, the condition of the patient, the availability of the burn team, and the desires of the patient.

Superficial partial thickness burns heal within 3 weeks and generally heal without hypertrophic scarring or major cosmetic deformity. Deep partial thickness burns take over 3 weeks to heal and may heal with hypertrophic scarring and significant cosmetic and functional problems.

Depth of the Burn Wound

The classical superficial partial thickness burn and the classical full thickness burn may be relatively easy to diagnose, but, for many burn injuries, the accurate diagnosis of the depth of injury is very difficult. Even the most experienced burn surgeons have much difficulty in accurately defining the depth of injury upon initial injury and there is no reliable laboratory test or device that consistently, and reliably measures physiological depth of injury. The burn depth of these injuries is therefore called indeterminate.

It is often advantageous to allow wounds to heal for 10 to 14 days so that a more accurate diagnosis of burn depth can be made. At that time, if the wound appears it will heal in another 7 to 10 days, then the wound is a superficial partial thickness burn wound and should do well without surgical intervention. If the wound appears that it will take longer than 10 days to heal, then the wound is a deep partial thickness and may benefit from surgical excision and wound closure.

Deep partial thickness burn injuries may take many weeks to become epithelialized. The few epithelial remnants in the wound produce epithelium and contraction occurs from the wound edges. The time to complete healing depends upon the thickness of the skin, the number of remaining epithelial appendages and the presence or absence of infection and/ or desiccation. These wounds generally benefit from early excision and wound closure to reduce the functional and cosmetic impairment.

Full thickness injuries can only heal by contraction of the wound edges which takes many weeks and months. This process may produce great deformity with hypertrophic scarring, contractures, and cosmetic impairment. Surgical excision and wound closure as early as possible is recommended.

Most burn injuries are not completely one depth of injury, but are a combination or mix of different depths of injury. Often times there will be a deep partial thickness or full thickness injury in the middle of the wound and superficial partial thickness injury around the edge. For patients with large total body surface areas involved, complex decisions are required to determine which areas to excise and which not to excise to obtain the maximum results. It is often best to treat an entire burned functional unit or aesthetic unit in the same manner. Burned units such as the dorsum of the hands, the arm, forearm, lower leg may be treated all the same with or without excision.

If mixed or combination depth injuries are present, it may be best to allow much of the wound to heal prior to excision of the smaller amount of surface area of the deep remaining wound. This allows for less total area requiring excision.

In general, burns which are deep partial thickness and full thickness injuries are good candidates for early surgical excisional therapy.

Etiology of the Burn Injury

The etiology of the burn injury is important because the depth of injury is closely related. Burns can be classified as flame/flash, scald, chemical, contact, and electrical. Scald burns can be from water or grease/oil. They may be from immersion or splash.

Chemical burns can be from acid, alkali, or petroleum products. Electrical burns can be high-voltage or low-voltage.

Deep burns are usually high-voltage electrical injuries, alkali and acid chemical injuries, immersion scalds, contact, and flame burns. Superficial burns are usually from flash injuries and water splashing scalding injuries. High-voltage electrical injuries usually require early surgical excision of all necrotic tissue, decompression of involved extremity compartments and early wound closure with grafts and/or flaps.

Location of the Burn

The location of the burn also must be considered in determining the advisability of surgical excision. The scalp has deep hair follicles which assist in epithelialization of the burn injury. It is preferable to allow maximum healing of the scalp rather than surgical excisional therapy because skin grafting of the scalp requires complex reconstruction methods to remove the skin graft secondarily. In addition the immobile scalp rarely produces hypertrophic scarring.

For combination of mixed injuries of the face, it is preferable to do late excision in aesthetic units to optimize results. The neck has very mobile skin and hypertrophic scarring often produces significant neck contractures; therefore surgical excisional therapy is often used to provide the best long term result with minimal contractures.

The dorsum of the hand is often involved in significant burns and does well with functional unit surgical excision of the burned area and wound closure. Deep burns to the volar hand and fingers are uncommon, but can be a major problem when they occur.

It is often best to excise the dorsum of the foot and toes to prevent extension contractures of the toes which prevent the wearing of shoes.

The back has thick skin and usually heals. In patients with large total body surface area burns, it is preferable to excise the back last because it often heals and the area is kept relatively clean because of the constant debriding action of patient movement on the sheets. The abdomen and breast are technically difficult to excise. Burns of the breast can produce contraction and displacement of the breast and/or the nipple/ areolar complex, therefore surgical excision and wound closure may alleviate the contraction processes.

General Condition of the Patient

The condition of the patient is important when considering excisional therapy. The patient must be medically stable prior to surgery. Any pre-existing diseases should be treated and the risks of surgical intervention must be weighed against the benefits. Often surgical therapy will be safer than non-surgical management.

Associated injuries must be noted and stabilized. Treatment of life threatening head, chest, and abdominal injuries take precedence over burn wound surgical excisional therapy. Bony fractures however may be managed concomitantly with burn excision.

Severe inhalation injury with unstable deteriorating pulmonary function is a contraindication to surgical excisional therapy until improvements occur. Coagulopathy, which is common after resuscitation of a major burn injury should be corrected before contemplating surgical excision.

Age of the Patient

Age is a relative consideration. The elderly have thinner skin from atrophy and injuries are commonly deep and require surgery. Their systemic reserves may be less and therefore may benefit the most from surgical excision and wound closure.

Timing of Excision

Once a diagnosis of the deep partial thickness or full thickness injury is made, then usually surgical excisional therapy should be accomplished as soon as the patient is stable and the operating room and operating team are available. For small deep burns, excision can be scheduled in the first few days.

For large deep burns, excision is usually accomplished within the first 5 days after injury. This does not allow heavy colonization of the burn wound with bacteria. Several trips to the operating room on multiple days may be necessary to completely excise the burn wound and obtain wound closure. A few burn centers practice excisional therapy within the first few hours of injury and note that the excision favorably influences the resuscitation phase. Certainly the patient must be stable prior to excisional therapy and we prefer that, excision after resuscitation is successfully completed.

Late surgical excision after 5 days can be utilized often times to optimize results. Patients with a large amount of the surface area of the wound noted to be indeterminate depth often benefit from waiting to see healing of the wound. It may take up to one to two weeks to accurately determine the depth of the wound. If the wound does not heal, then the patient is brought to surgery for excisional treatment.

In some patients wound depth is known, but a large surface area of the wound is superficial and a small surface area of the wound is deep. It may be advantageous to allow the superficial portion to heal prior to surgical excision of the deep portion. We prefer to wait 10-14 days to allow epithelialization in this type of injury.

For patients who have large total body surface area of deep burns, multiple trips to the operating room for staged excision and wound closure are necessary. These later procedures are late excisions but are necessary because of the massive amount of injured skin that must be excised.

General Guidelines for Excision

The techniques of surgical excision vary, but many guidelines have been established to help the surgeon. When patients have only small total body surface area burns, area requiring maximum functional and cosmetic results are the first priority. These areas are the hands, face, neck, and feet. Although some have advocated early excisional therapy of the face, most centers would wait 7-10 days and excise the face as aesthetic units. For patients with large total body surface area burns, other considerations may be involved. If depth is a major concern, many centers excise large surface areas of the burn as a first priority. This accomplishes removal of the most necrotic material and diminishes the risk of sepsis more than if only a small functional or aesthetic area were excised first. Therefore, areas such as the chest, abdomen, back, and legs are a priority, and hands face neck and feet are excised later. In general, an experienced burn surgical team should use staged surgical excisions for patients with over 30 percent burn. Excision should limit to no more than 20 percent of the total body surface area per operation. The procedure should not exceed 2 hours. The excision should not cause the loss of more than one unit of blood volume per operation. However up to 35 percent of the total body surface area can be excised if tourniquets are used for blood loss control. In addition always attempt to excise the deeper burns initially during the staged procedures.

The burn surgical team may consist of 2 or 3 teams of surgeons working on 2 or 3 different areas simultaneously to minimise the time under anesthesia. The burn excision sites should always be "closed" at the termination of the procedure with temporary or permanent techniques, described in the previous chapter.

Preparations for surgical excision are necessary to provide for safety and optimal results. Pre-operatively the surgical team should discuss the role of each member and the overall sequence of events to occur in the operating room. No time should be wasted in the operating room to discuss strategies, if the decisions can be made pre-operatively. Blood availability must be assured prior to the incision and infusions may need to be started prior to the incisions. Intravenous access and arterial monitoring lines should be placed immediately prior to surgery. Plans should be made for wound closure, either temporary or permanent, pre-operatively. The status of the wound should be determined and excisional therapy and wound closure should only be performed on minimally colonized wounds. Wound biopsies may be helpful in this determination.

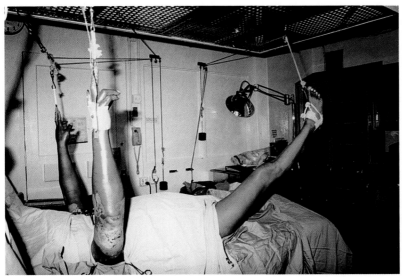

Figure 8.1: Elevation of extremities by hanging from a specially constructed frame on the ceiling and counter-traction with weights on pulleys. This system helps to change the angle of elevation for easy access on the limb circumferentially for wound excision, skin harvesting, control blood loss and application of skin grafts

Surgical teams, operating suite and all needed personnel must be available for the procedure. Antibiotics specific for the wound flora or broad spectrum antibiotics are usually given peri-operatively.

Preparations are made to allow for optimal positioning of the patient in surgery. For the extremities, hooks extending from the ceiling are helpful to hang gently the arm or leg for excision (Figure 8.1). The head and scalp may require specialized devices to expose all burned areas. Patient warmth must be maintained with operating room ambient temperature above 80°F, warm blankets, fluids, and sterile warm sheets during surgery.

Bleeding must be controlled with pressure, elevation, topical thrombin, epinephrine solution and application of skin grafts.

METHODS OF EXCISION

The surgical excision of the burn wound can be accomplished by a tangential technique or fascial technique. Each technique has its own advantages and disadvantages.

TANGENTIAL EXCISION

When first reported by Janzekovic, the technique of tangential excision actually presented three controversial concepts: (l)That the deep partial burn wounds should be excised early. (2) that they could be excised with preservation of some dermal elements and (3) Wound bed with dermal elements permit graft take. These ideas are now all widely accepted largely due to the success of tangential or "layered" excision of partial and full-thickness burns (Figures 8.2A to C).

As outlined by Jackson, burn wounds consists of a central area of coagulation necrosis surrounded by a zone of capillary stasis and an outer layer of hyperemia (See chapter on anatomy of the Burn Wound). Under ordinary circumstances that is, in the absence of infection, the hyperemic zone is alive and quickly heals while the zone of necrosis is dead and sloughs. The zone of stasis is more complex: Left alone, it takes on an appearance identical to that of coagulation necrosis and will usually slough as well. This zone contains necrotic epidermal elements but also has patent capillaries. Janzekovic demonstrated that excision to this level exposes a layer of punctate bleeding that will take skin grafts well despite the presence of some non-viable tissue. In deep partial-thickness burns, this layer also contains dermal collagen which, when preserved, appears to minimize scarring following grafting, producing a better cosmetic and functional result than similar wounds which are permitted to heal on their own.

Technique

The wound is excised with large (Watson/Humby) or small Goulian hand-held dermatomes or with powered dermatomes set to remove eschar at a thickness of 0.010-0.20 inches. Sequential passes are made over a particular area, and the bed inspected after each pass. The end point of excision is the presence of uniform punctate bleeding. Any non-bleeding areas must be re-excised. If excision is carried out under tourniquet, any areas of reddish-discolored tissue are removed, leaving a base of waxy-white dermis or, in full-thickness

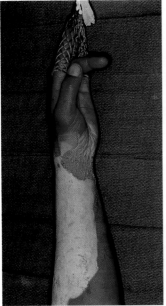
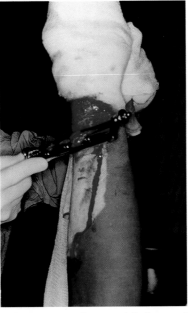

Figure 8.2A: Elevation of fore-arm and hand in preparation for the burn wound excision

Figure 8.2B: Sequential (layered) excision of the deep burn wound

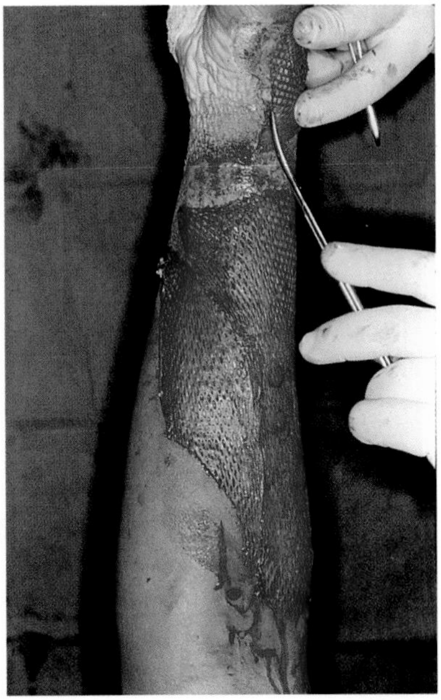

Figure 8.2C: Application of skin grafts after excision and achieving haemo-stasis

burns, pale yellow subcutaneous fat. At the completion of excision, the tourniquet is released briefly to check for the presence of uniform bleeding. Since wounds which are excised in this manner bleed heavily, it is advisable to perform skin grafting in a separate procedure.

Indication for Sequential (Layered) Excision

1. All excisions of partial-thickness burns.
2. Excision of mixed second and third-degree burns.
3. Excision of full-thickness burn where the subcutaneous fat is sufficiently vascularized to permit graft take (hands, face, etc.). In most patients, almost all excisions can be done to this level with success. Exceptions are the elderly and the obese.
4. Excision of burns where preservation of subcutaneous contours is important. Examples include the hand, the face, the breast, and small burns where fascial excision would create an unacceptable defect.
5. Excision of burns of questionable depth. A single pass taken at a depth of .08-0.10 inches reveals whether the wound needs to be grafted or not.

Contraindications

1. Blood loss: Layered excisions results in more blood loss than fascial excisions. This limits the size of a single procedure to about 20 percent TBSA. In very bloody areas i.e. the face, subcutaneous infiltration of epinephrine can help control blood loss.

2. Layered excisions of large areas take longer than fascial excisions. Layered excisions of full-thickness burns can produce a graft bed with poor blood supply. The abdomen, thigh, upper arm, etc. have deep, "lumpy" subcutaneous fat which may not take a graft well. Judgment is necessary in deciding whether to continue excision deeper. However, we usually begin with layered excision since it is always possible to go deeper. Layered excisions of old or separating eschar are technically difficult. Layered excisions may not be appropriate for septic wounds.

PRIMARY OR FULL FASCIAL EXCISION

Traditionally, grafting onto fascia or muscle has been favored over grafting onto fat in patients with full-thickness burns. This concept of preferential grafting onto fascia is based on several clinical impressions: Firstly, that fat is less resistant to trauma and more susceptible to secondary infections than fascia. Secondly, that excision to fascia is associated with less bleeding than excision to fat. Lastly, that grafts placed on fat will have a higher percentage of graft loss than grafts placed on fascia. However, the routine application of fascial excision of deep burns may result in unnecessary cosmetic disfigurement and lead to the development of more severe lymphedema and contractures in patients with circumferential extremity burns. Based on a prospective study of the effect of the recipient bed on skin graft survival after thermal injury (Deitch in 1985 demonstrated that in patients with burns <60 percent TBSA, there is no advantage to routinely performing fascial excision to avoid grafting onto fat. This conclusion is based on a mean graft take of 94 percent on fat versus 85 percent on fascia (p=0.21).

However, there are some patients in whom grafting directly onto fascia is appropriate. One group includes patients with massive (>60% TBSA) burns in whom widely meshed skin grafts are used since, skin grafts placed on fat are more susceptible to delayed loss due to desiccation than grafts placed on fascia or muscle. A second group of patients in whom grafting onto fascia is favored are patients with combined surface burns and inhalation injuries, since these patients are at an increased risk of developing septic complications. Grafts placed on fat are more susceptible to secondary loss than grafts placed on fascia, if the patient becomes septic.

The question of whether to graft on fat or fascia must be individualized in elderly patients, patients on steroids, and patients with connective tissue disorders, since in these patients, graft loss is potentially higher when fat is used as the recipient bed for the skin graft due to impaired cutaneous blood flow. As a rule of thumb, one should prefer fascia over fat as the graft bed of choice in individuals in whom graft loss would jeopardize survival.

Technique

Primary or fascial excision is performed by grasping the burn eschar with towel clips and then using the Bovie electrocautery to excise the burned tissue by traction-avulsion and cutting (Figure 8.3). The use of the electrocautery minimizes blood loss and speeds up the procedure (Figures 8.4A and B).

In summary, surgical excisional therapy of the burn wound is an accepted method of care for the treatment of selected cases of patients with deep burn injuries. Most centers feel

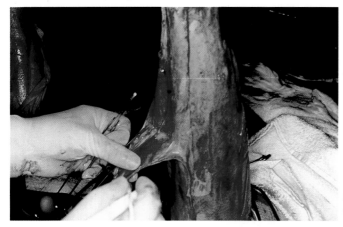

Figure 8.3: Primary (fascial) excision of the leg with traction avulsion of the eschar and using electrocautery for cutting

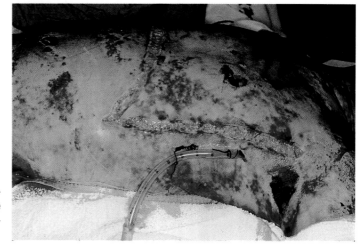

Figure 8.4A: Circumferential full- thickness burns of the trunk with chest tube for pneumothorax and chest escharotomies in a 43 year old male

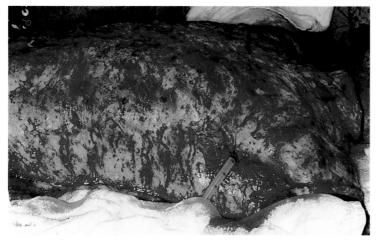

Figure 8.4B: Primary excision of deep burns of the neck, chest wall, abdomen up to the groin and extending laterally to the posterior axillary line on both sides

patients with small burns of less than 20 percent total body surface area can be safely excised with a decrease in hospital stay, less costs, and less time away from home, work, and school.

The pain of the injury can be diminished with surgical excision and wound closure. In selected cases, there can be functional and cosmetic improvement with surgical excision and wound closure. With newer techniques of wound closure, there may be better survival rates in patients with large burns over 70 percent of body surface.

BIBLIOGRAPHY

1. Baxter CR, Curreri PW, Heimbach DM *et al: Manual of Excision*: a compilation from the excision roundtable at the third Maui Burn Conference, Maui, Hawaii, January 1988.
2. Boswick J Jr (Ed): *The Art and Science of Burn Care*, Aspen Publishers, Inc., Rockville, Maryland, 255-262, 1987.
3. Burke JF, Bondoci CC, Quinby WC: Primary burn excision and immediate grafting, a method of shortening illness. *J Trauma* 14:389-395, 1974.
4. Deitch EA: A Policy of early excision and grafting in elderly burn patients shortens the hospital stay and improves survival. *Burns* **12 (2):** 109-114, 1985.
5. Heimbach DM: Early burn excsion and grafting, in burns, the Surgical Clinics of North America. WB Saunders Co., Philadelphia, **67 (1):** 96-107, 1987.
6. Heimbach DM, Engrav LH (Eds): *Surgical Management of the Burn Wound*. Raven Press, New York, 1984.
7. Herndon D, Gore D, Cole M *et al:* Determinants of mortality in pediatric patients with greater than 70% full-thickness total body surface area thermal injury treated by early excision and grafting. *J Trauma* 27:208, 1987.
8. Jackson D, Mac G: Second thoughts on the burn wound. *J Trauma* **9:**839- 862, 1969.
9. Jackson DM, Stone PA: Tangential excision and grafting of burn- the method, and report of 50 consecutive cases. *Br J Plast Surg* **25:** 416-426, 1972.
10. Janzekovic Z: A new concept in the early excision and immediate grafting of burns. *J Trauma* **10:**1103-1108, 1970.
11. Merrell SW, Saffle JR, Sullivan JJ *et al:* Increased survival after major thermal injury: a nine-year review. *Amer J Surg* **154:**623-627,1987
12. Tompkins RG, Schoenfeld DA, Gehringer GC *et al:* Prompt eschar excison: a treatment system contibuting to reduced burn mortality. *Ann Surg* **204:** 272-281, 1986.

9

Management of Burn Wounds in Special Areas

The location of burn wounds in special anatomical areas creates a unique problem. Surgical or nonsurgical management of these burns needs special attention.

BURNS OF THE SCALP

Scalp burns can be associated with thermal, chemical or electrical injuries. The depth of burn wounds to the scalp can range from superficial partial thickness burns to injuries involving cranium.

Scalp burn wounds are frequently associated with other extensive burn injuries, else where on the body which may require major surgical procedures. Therefore, a simple effective treatment of burns is important in the overall management of burned patients.

Based on anatomical considerations and according to the extent and depth of the burn wound, the following simple guidelines will help the clinician in the management. Because of the rich blood supply and the presence of numerous skin appendages, superficial and even deep dermal scalp burns, of any extent can readily epithelialize and should be treated conservatively. Full thickness scalp burns should be surgically excised. One should wait ten days to two weeks before excision, in order to give time for the partial thickness wound to heal. The excision should be carried deep into the subdermal tissue and should include all remaining skin appendages before applying a split thickness skin graft **(Figures 9.1A to C)**. Otherwise, they may form inclusion cysts, or subsequent hair growth may promote secondary graft loss. Necrotic or non-viable soft tissue in subdermal burns can be debrided, but pericranium should always be preserved, so that a skin graft can be applied. The secondary alopecia can be corrected at a later date with tissue expansion. If the skull bones are denuded over a surface area less than half of the scalp, a local transposed or rotational flap is then the preferred method of coverage **(Figures 9.2A to C)**. The necrotic bone acts as a bone graft and eventually gets absorbed under a vascular flap.

If more than half of the skull is exposed with no viable pericranium, then the outer table of the skull should be excised to expose the vascular dipole, so that a split thickness skin graft can be applied immediately **(Figures 9.3A to F)**. Free flaps or distant pedicle flaps are rarely indicated and should be avoided in this acute setting.

By following this simple algorithm **(Chart 9.1)** of surgical management, subdermal burn wounds of the scalp can be closed early and effectively.

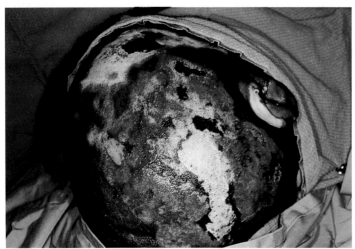

Figure 9.1A: Full thickness and deep partial thickness burns of the scalp

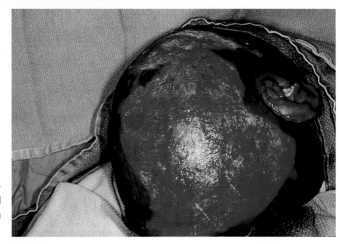

Figure 9.1B: Sequential excision performed on 10th postburn day and wound covered with meshed split thickness skin grafts

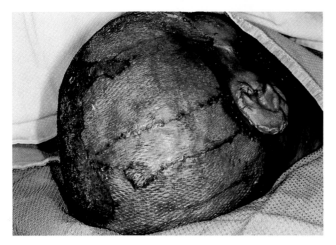

Figure 9.1C: Healed wound with complete graft take 7 days after surgery

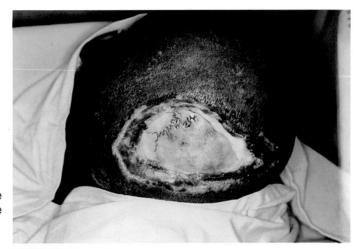

Figure 9.2A: Electrical contact burn of the scalp with involvement of the outer table of the skull

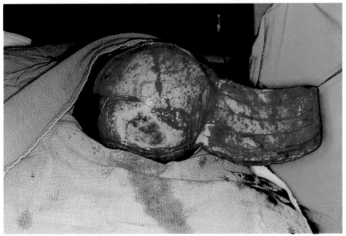

Figure 9.2B: After triangular excision of the wound, a temperoparietal transposed skin flap raised. Note the longitudinal incisions in the galea along the long axis of the flap to increase the width of the flap and easy insertion without tension

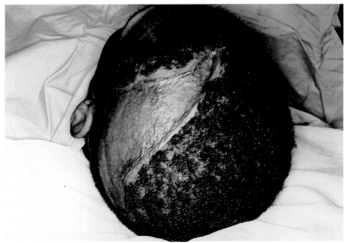

Figure 9.2C: Final result 2 months after surgery

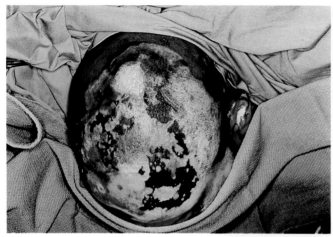

Figure 9.3A: Deep burns involving two-thirds of the scalp

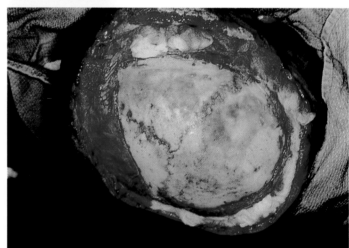

Figure 9.3B: Wounds after surgical excision one week after, exposing the outer table of the scalp over large area

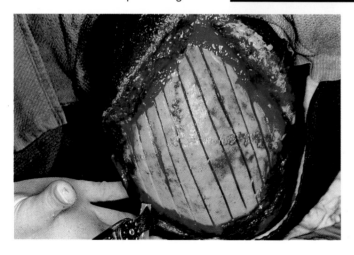

Figure 9.3C: Grid incisions are made with electric saw in preparation for excision of the outer table

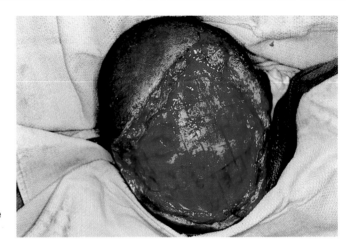

Figure 9.3D: Excision of the outer table completed, exposing the vascular diploe

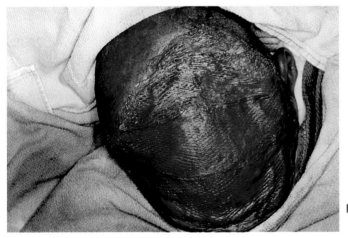

Figure 9.3E: Vascular diploe covered with meshed split thickness skin grafts

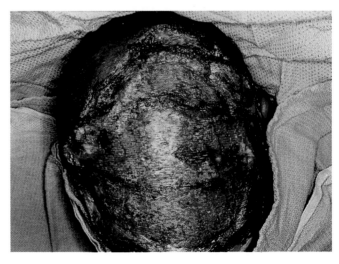

Figure 9.3F: Two weeks after surgery showing complete graft take and wound healing

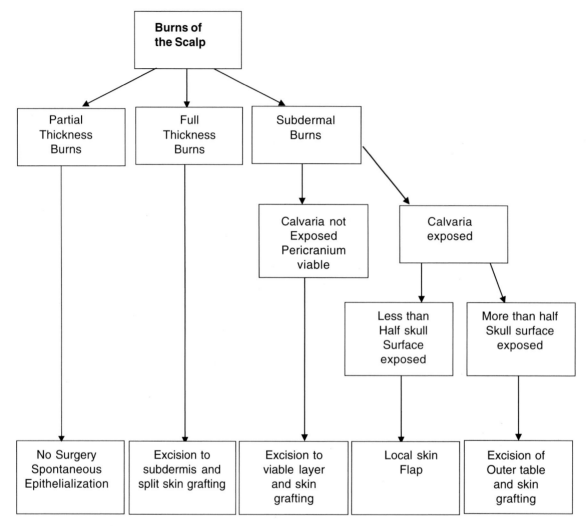

Chart 9.1: Algorithm of surgical management of deep burns of the scalp

BURNS OF THE FACE

Burns of the face and particularly of the specialized structures including eyelids, nose and ears pose unique wound management considerations. These burns should ideally be treated in a specialized burn care facility. The goal is to preserve the tissue from infection and encourage rapid uncomplicated healing, leading to optimal function and aesthetic recovery.

Wound Care

In addition to the general care described in the chapter on the initial care of the burn wound, the following principles for the care of facial burns are important.

1. Gentle cleaning with saline or hydrotherapy.
2. Q-Tip cleaning of nasal orifices.
3. Shaving of facial and proximal scalp hair involved in burn injury, however eyebrows and eyelashes must be preserved.
4. Application of topical antimicrobial ointment and covering it with Vaseline gauze or fine mesh gauze dressings.
5. Change dressings once or twice per day or alternatively treat by open method with frequent application of ointment or cream.

Lips and tip of the nose should be treated with frequent application of ointment and aggressive debridement of crusts should be avoided. Daily shaving of the face is recommended regardless of depth of injury. Meticulous oral hygiene must be practiced daily.

Because of the rich vascularity, facial burns heal very quickly. Deep burns that take more than three weeks to close result in ugly scars and disfigurement. Full thickness burns need early excision and grafting. Deep burns should be initially treated conservatively with daily hydrotherapy, debridement and topical antimocrobials. Very superficial burns can be covered with porcine xenografts or other biological dressings. On day ten, the burn wounds should be evaluated in determining which areas are not healed and will not be healed with in three weeks of burn injury for planning excision and grafting.

Method of Excision and Grafting of Facial Burns

The operation is carried out under general anesthesia with the patient in the reverse Trendelenburg position. Ace bandages should be applied on the lower extremities to prevent venous stasis. Intradental wire fixation of the endotracheal tube will help to secure the tube with full access to the face. Contact lenses may be used to protect the cornea. Those aesthetic units judged to be incapable of healing with in three weeks of the injury are out lined with a marker. Frequently small unburned or healed areas must be included in the excision to preserve the aesthetic unit **(Figure 9.4A)**.

The goulian knife with a 0.008 inch guard is used for the excision and that is continued until normal tissue is visualized. If superficial areas are included in the unit, they need to be excised deeply enough to prevent the wound from healing underneath the graft, resulting in secondary graft loss. When excising the eyelids, three traction stitches are placed in the lid margin and used to place tension on the lids. Hemostasis is achieved with electrocoagulation and epinephrine (1:10,000) soaked gauze pads **(Figure 9.4B)**. The excised areas are then covered with sheet auto graft of 0.018-0.025 inches in thickness. If the hemostasis is not too satisfactory, the excised areas are then covered with allograft with all that attention one would give to autografts. Usually with in forty-eight hours the patient is returned to the operating room for autografting. The split thickness skin grafts are usually obtained from the scalp if one must match graft color with the color of healed or unburned areas. If the entire face is to be grafted, color match becomes a problem except that the entire face should be of the same color. In the latter situation, the grafts may be obtained wherever adequate skin is available. However it is generally unwise to obtain these thick grafts from upper chest or neck in women, since the donor sites tend to develop hypertrophic scarring. The graft is then carefully stitched into place in the aesthetic units **(Figure 9.4C)**. Dressings are applied and fixed with pressure garments, elastomere or orthoplast splints.

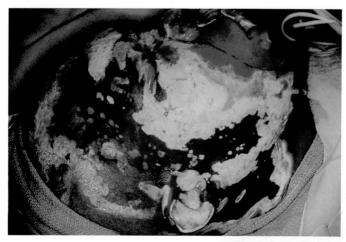

Figure 9.4A: Full thickness burns of the face. Note that the marking of surgical excision included a small unburned area near the nasolabial fold

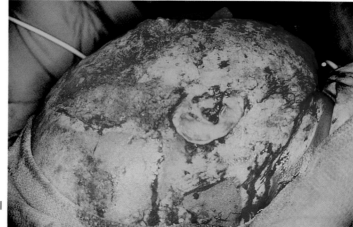

Figure 9.4B: Facial burns, after surgical excision and complete hemostasis

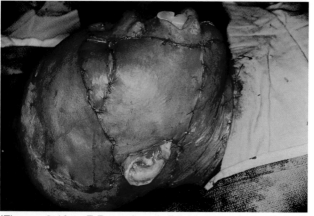

Figure 9.4C: Excised wounds are covered with thick split thickness skin grafts, placed in aesthetic units and sutured in place

(Figures 9.4A to F Reproduced with kind permission from Dr. Thatte, Editor of the "Indian Journal of Plastic Surgery," December 1988. Volume 21. No. 2: "Recent Trends in Management of Burns" by Marella L. Hanumadass, Page 80-81, Fig. 6-9)

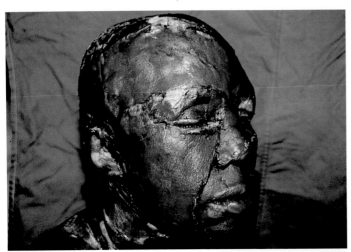

Figure 9.4D: Appearance of the grafts on 5th postoperative day at the 1st dressing change

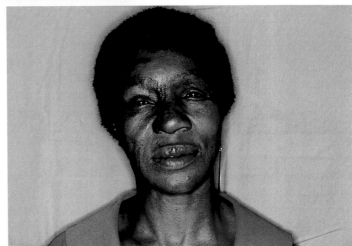

Figure 9.4E: Postoperative appearance 6 months after grafting

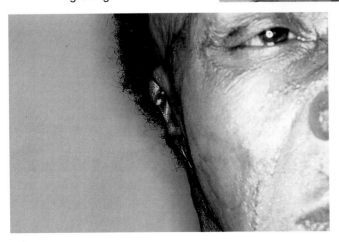

Figure 9.4F: Closeup view of the grafts

Postoperatively the grafts are inspected and any hematomas removed through one centimeter incisions placed in the relaxed skin tension lines. Patients are kept on nil per mouth (NPO) for three days and encouraged to refrain from talking. Inter maxillary fixation to achieve total immobilization is usually not indicated (Figures 9.4D to F).

BURN OF THE PERIORBITAL REGION

Eyelid burns occur in 8 to 27% of all patients with major burn injuries and in 18 to 67% of patients presenting with facial burns. The most common sequelae of eyelid burns are lid retraction or ectropion. Inadequate treatment of eyelid burns and the ensuing lid retraction may result in chronic conjunctivitis, keratitis, or corneal ulceration, with ultimate permanent visual impairment. Therefore, timely and aggressive treatment is essential.

Most superficial partial thickness eyelid burns will heal spontaneously without functional impairment with simple local treatment i.e. superficial debridement, wound cleaning and corneal protection. However, many deep partial thickness and all full thickness burns will need additional measures in order to restore and preserve normal lid function. Three to 12% of all facial burns result in ectropion and 10 to 45% of these ectropion will be of such severity that operative correction is required (Figures 9.5A to C).

However in most partial thickness severe facial burns with edema the lids are closed for several days, naturally protecting the cornea.

With improved resuscitative measures, more patients are surviving previously lethal burns. Consequently, the optimal treatment is to restore normal long term function to burned eyelids.

The lower eyelid is relatively immobile and initial edema protects the globe of the eye in acute stage. In a series of 124 eyelid Burns reported by Ash et al, the earliest onset of lower eyelid ectropion was three weeks postburn (Range of three to seventeen weeks). This delayed and protracted lid retraction exposes the globe. The presence of ectropion is not itself an indication for immediate surgery, if there are other reconstructive priorities. Release of the lid and inlay thick split thickness grafting should be done if there is chronic conjunctivitis or lack of a positive bell's phenomenon and danger of corneal damage. Often the upper and the lower lids are involved resulting in severe lid shortening, which forces the surgeons to correct the defect earlier.

Until recently, the most commonly used techniques for treatment of severe eyelid burns involved tarsorrhaphy or other means of forced lid closure and immobilization. Much of the early approach to treating eyelid burns was derived from experiences with nonthermal eyelid trauma. It is important to note that there are essential differences between burn injuries and eyelid injuries due to other mechanisms. Eyelid lacerations or avulsions often result in full thickness loss of tissue extending from skin to conjuctiva, which sometimes include loss of the tarsal plate. In these instances, functional lid closure and globe coverage often requires a tarsal bridging procedure or tarsorrhaphy.

In contrast to nonthermal eyelid trauma, eyelid burns result in lid retraction or shortened lid excursion due to contraction of the burned skin. Due to reflexive blinking and tight eyelid closure when the patient is exposed to flame or caustic materials, the ciliary margins and deeper structures, i.e. tarsal plate are usually preserved.

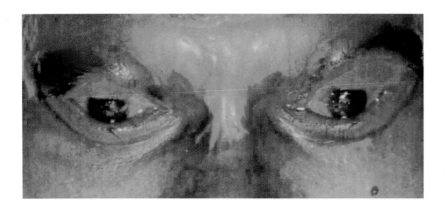

Figure 9.5A: Healed burns of the face and periorbital region showing ectropion of both the upper eyelids

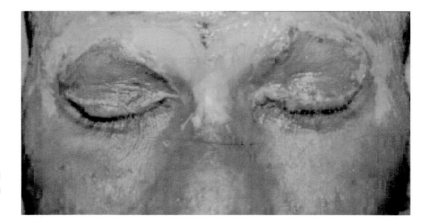

Figure 9.5B: After correction of the ectropion and skin grafting with eyes open

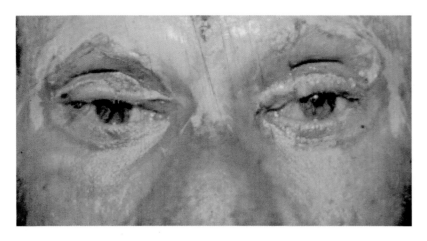

Figure 9.5C: Same patient with eyes closed

If tarsorrhaphy is performed on a burned, retracted eyelid, the closure will often be under tension. If the stitches around the tarsal plate are under tension, perfusion of the lid margin and tarsal plate will be impaired. This may result in permanent distortion of the lid margin or necrosis of the tarsal plate. Furthermore, examination of the globe and the application of ophthalmic medications are difficult after tarsorrhaphy and if both eyes are closed simultaneously, the prolonged visual obstruction may have unfavorable psychological effects on the convalescing burn patients.

In case of a deep upper eyelid and forehead burn, intrinsic contraction of the burned eyelids results in foreshortening and tightening of the eschar bands in both horizontal and vertical direction. The vertical retraction is further exacerbated by the upward traction transmitted by the contracting forehead eschar. Thus, significant eyelid retraction and immobility, accelerated by the forehead eschar, become evident as early as the third postburn day.

In addition, to the lid retraction, the prolapse of the swollen conjunctiva further complicates the problem. The precise etiology of the conjunctival prolapse is not clear, but it may be assumed that the inelastic, lid which is stretched tightly from medial to lateral canthus, produces a tourniquet effect, thereby compromising the venous and lymphatic efflux from the conjunctiva; the palpebral and bulbar conjunctival edema progresses while the eyelid remained tightly retracted, resulting in the obliteration of the superior fornix. Ultimately, the conjuctiva prolapsed from under the shortened eyelid becomes irreducible. The regular application of protective ointments to the conjuctiva is only a temporary measure.

The iminent risk of exposure and injury to the conjunctiva and the globe require early therapeutic intervention with eyelid escharotomy and immediate skin grafting technique (Figures 9.6A to F). Superciliary incision is made on the upper eyelid extending 5 mm beyond the lateral and medial canthi. The incision should be carried down to the palpebral conjunctiva so that the strangulating tension imposed by the tight eschar bands across the upper eyelids are relieved. Temporary sutures may be placed along the ciliary lid margin for traction and stabilization of the lid. The margin of the upper eyelid can be advanced now to a level well below the lower lid margin. The edematous prolapsed conjunctiva can also be reduced to normal anatomic position, restoring the previously obliterated superior fornix. Split thickness skin graft should be inlayed immediately and secured to the eyelid with interrupted 0-5 silk stitches around the perimeter of that defect. The end of the tied sutures may be used to fasten a stented dressing.

There is some controversy as to the best type of graft for deep eyelid burns and to optimal time of eschar excision and grafting. The majority of authors recommend a split thickness skin graft for coverage of upper eyelid burns and full thickness graft for lower eyelid. Some authors advocate the use of full thickness grafts for upper lids, suggesting that this lowers the propensity for late contracture and ectropion. The split thickness type graft has the advantages of remaining supple and being easier to procure than a full-thickness graft. Split thickness grafts have functioned well with excellent graft viability in our experience.

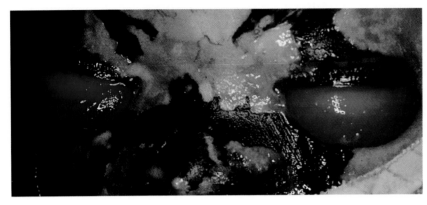

Figure 9.6A: 18-month old African American female with full thickness burns to her forehead, eyelids, and nose. Notice prolapse of the palpebral conjunctiva of the upper eyelids with complete obliteration of the superior fornix

Figure 9.6B: Same patient with superciliary incision of the upper eyelid, exposing the palpebral conjunctiva. The incisions extended beyond the medial and lateral canthus

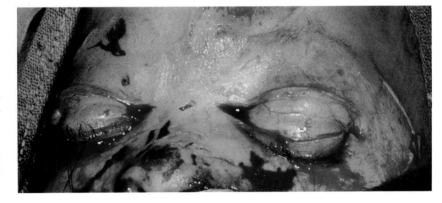

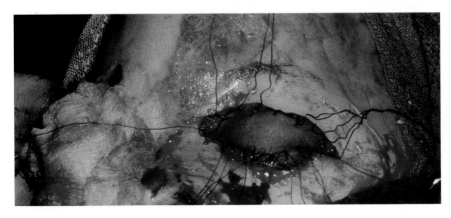

Figure 9.6C: Split thickness skin graft placed onto wound bed and sutured in place

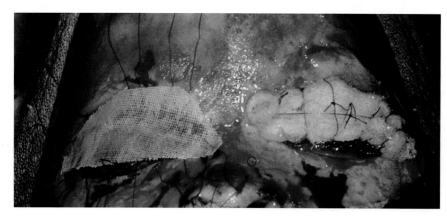

Figure 9.6D: Stented dressing in place to fix the graft and immobilize the eyelids

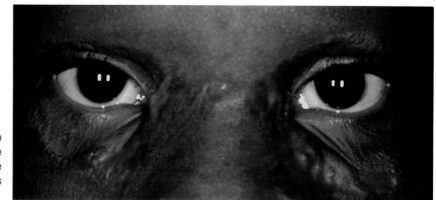

Figure 9.6E: This two year follow up picture illustrates the graft on the upper eyelids, with eyes open

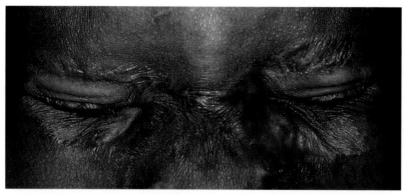

Figure 9.6F: Two year follow up, demonstrating full function of the upper eyelids with no further corrective surgery with eye closed

BURN INJURY TO THE EAR

Direct thermal injury of the ear may vary from mere erythema of the skin to desiccation of the cartilage and resulting complications. One tends to ignore the ear, while treating an otherwise severe deep burn, and finally realize that the ear burn takes the longest time to heal. Desiccation of the cartilage may result in sloughing and necrosis of the entire ear. The pattern of the burn wound in the ear has to be carefully watched, so as to plan the treatment. Ear burn also is one where priority treatment must be given and also individualized.

The anatomy of the external ear has to be recapitulated. This consists of conchal cartilage with folds and depressions, over which full thickness skin is snugly wrapped. Between the skin and the cartilage, there is a layer of areolar tissue also. The skin is also nonhair bearing. The cartilage consists of yellow elastic fibers covered with peri chondrium. The lobule of the ear is soft, does not contain cartilage but consists of fibro fatty tissue. The cartilage of the auricle is prolonged inwards in a tubular fashion as the cartilage of the external auditory meatus, whose attachment to the bone, stabilizes the auricle in position.

Etiological Factors

Thermal burn is the most common injury. Scalding occurs as part of the generalized burning. Acid burns occur usually as a part of homicidal injury and electrical burns though rare, do occur. Sometimes Xray therapy to the cervical glands may cause radiation burn of the ear.

Clinical Presentation

Superficial burn: This appears as an area of erythema, with evidence of edema and swelling and minute bleeding may be noticed. Even without any active treatment, the lesion will heal. But as the superficial burn is very painful, Analgesics and other topical soothing creams may be used. Full thickness burns of the skin of the ear usually looks dark, depressed without evidence of edema. Commonly in less serious cases the margins of the helix are affected. But if the entire skin is affected with deep burn, invariably the cartilage also gets affected, and the ear looks parchment like at this stage. All measures have to be taken to protect the cartilage. If the perichondrium can be preserved, split thickness skin graft can be applied after removing the dead skin carefully under anesthesia.

Two types of thermal damage to the external ear can occur. The first is a full thickness burn of the ear where the cartilage is directly involved. Most commonly affected areas are helix and anti helix, though the entire ear may be involved. Sometimes if the injury is severe auto amputation of the pinna occurs. If the injury is not severe, the marginal necrotic area and the eschar separates by itself and the rest of the area heals without infection. The auto chondrectomy is a term that has been used to describe this process. This process does leave a severe deformity. The second type of auricular damage is the suppurative chondritis, where secondary infection damages the cartilage. It occurs as a late phenomenon after 3 to 6 weeks postburn. Auricular cartilage is especially vulnerable to injury owing to its exposed position and lack of subcutaneous tissue between skin and the perichondrium. It is interesting to note that suppurative chondritis develops in superficial and deep partial thickness injuries, which gets infected. The exposed cartilage and full thickness burns never develop chrondritis.

This is because the cartilage is totally avascular and devoid of perichondrium in full thickness burn. In superficial and deep partial thickness burns, the organisms first infect the skin, perichondrium and enter the cartilage.

The non-viable cartilage is a potential nidus for bacterial colonization and sepsis. Clinically suppurative chondritis once sets in progresses rapidly. The ear gets swollen, edematous, the healthy skin if any shows edema, and is very tender to touch. Inflammation starts on the helix and anti helix or the tragus and spread to other areas. Finally the infection results in an abscess formation,

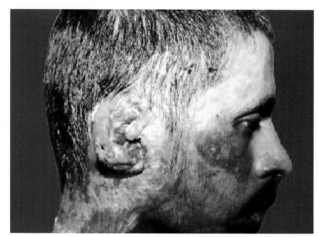

Figure 9.7: Chondritis

which either empties by itself or can be, incised **(Figures 9.7 and 9.8A to C)**. The necrosed cartilage comes out as purulent material. Finally after all the necrotic material comes out, the ear shrinks into a cauliflower shape and consists of only skin on either side filled with fibrous tissue.

Management

The important principle in the management of burnt ear is to prevent pressure, which may aggravate any existing burn. If both sides of the ears are involved, carefully prepared plastic cups are placed over the ear and are fixed by adhesives **(Figure 9.9)**. Even if the patient turns to one side and lies down, the ear cannot get pressure damage.

If the burn is full thickness, and if cartilage can be saved, the dead skin is excised and the perichondrium is covered with split thickness skin graft. In partial thickness burns, dressings are done daily and topical antimicrobial cream-like silver sulfadiazine is applied.

Occasionally iontophoresis with topical antibiotics can also be used to prevent skin necrosis.

When suppurative chrondritis and abscess occurs, careful bivalving along the helical margin is done and purulent matter is scooped out and pressure dressings are used on either side of the ear. This type of treatment will prevent crippling deformity of the ear. Once the wound heals, it will be easier to reconstruct the framework either by auto cartilage or by synthetic implants. Timely intervention would help to preserve the skin of the ear.

ACUTE HAND BURNS

The hand is the most frequently injured area of the body. The hands are burned in nearly 50% of patients admitted to burn centers. Whether part of a larger burn or hand burn alone. Burn injuries of the hands require an organized, thorough and systematic approach in order to provide the basis for a successful outcome. Frequently however, despite the best treatment regimens,

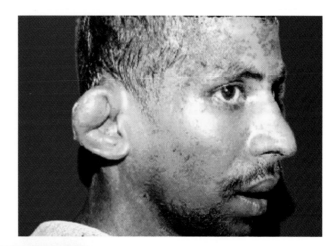

Figure 9.8A: Chondral abscess

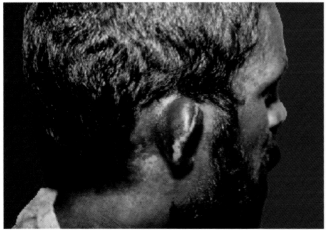

Figure 9.8B: Bivalving of the pinna

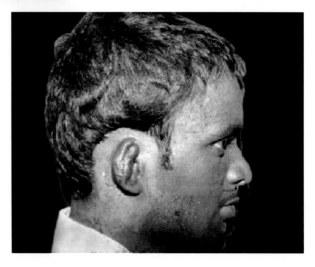

Figure 9.8C: Final result

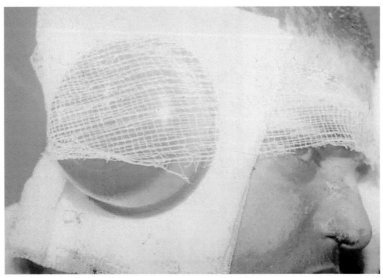

Figure 9.9: Protective dressing

the severity of the injury precludes optimal functional return. Nevertheless, adherence of basic principles of management at the initiation of treatment may significantly reduce long term morbidity and improve functional results. Initial assessment should include a detailed history and physical examination. Extent of injury, depth of injury and neurovascular status should be carefully evaluated and documented. Secondary evaluation everyday is essential.

Initial Wound Care

The wounds are cleaned and debrided (see the chapter on the Initial Care of the Burn Wound) and covered with antimicrobial cream. Very superficial burns may be covered with biological dressings. Control of edema during emergency and acute phase is very important otherwise, it may lead to fibrosis and ischemic necrosis of the intrinsic muscles of the hand. The elevation of the hand should be at heart level. If the elbow is not affected it could be flexed at 90° and placed in a sling. Prolonged elbow flexion may result in increasing internal pressure, so elbow extension and elevation of the extremity utilizing pillows should also be instituted.

Exercise

The physical and occupational therapists should immediately become involved in managing the burns of the hand, because even short delays can cause permanent damage or prolong the recovery of joints, tendons, ligaments and skin. Important points in exercising the hand include:
1. Muscle contraction should be forceful enough to serve as a pumping mechanism to help venous blood and lymph return
2. Passive range of motion and stretching may lead to further injury
3. Exercise should be done during dressing changes
4. Involvement of the patient in age appropriate activities.

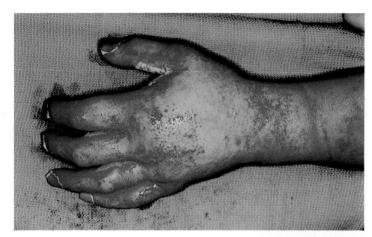

Figure 9.10A: Deep partial thickness burns, dorsum of the hand

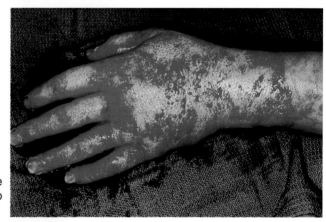

Figure 9.10B: Tangential excision up to the level of punctate bleeding. Note that the deep viable dermal tissue is preserved

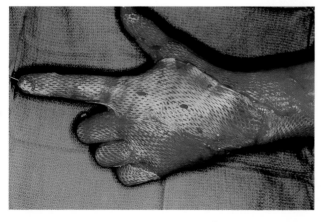

Figure 9.10C: 1:1.5 Meshed split thickness skin grafts placed to cover the excised wound. The meshed grafts are placed without spreading

(Figures 9.10A to D Reproduced with kind permission from Dr. Thatte, Editor of the "Indian Journal of Plastic Surgery," December 1988. Volume 21. No. 2: "Recent Trends in Management of Burns" by Marella L. Hanumadass, Page 80, Fig. 2-6)

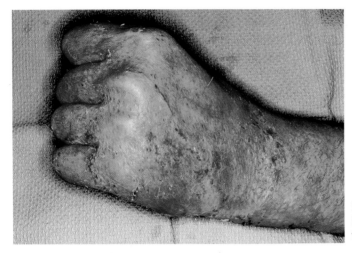

Figure 9.10D: On postoperative day 10, hand showing complete graft take and full function of the hand

Early surgical wound closure of hand burns: Every effort should be made to close the deep burns of the hand by early surgical excision and grafting.

Localized deep partial thickness burns on the dorsum of the hand can be tangentially excised within 72 hours and covered with split thickness skin grafts **(Figures 9.10A to D)**. The hand should be immobilized in functional position with splints and elevated postoperatively.

Full thickness burns can also be excised sequentially and closed with skin grafts. It is better to do excision under tourniquet to preserve the paratenon and neurovascular structures on the volar aspect of the hand and thick split thickness skin grafts (0.020"-0.025") are used to cover the wounds **(Figures 9.11A to C)**. If the joints are exposed, an internal or external fixation may be contemplated. If tendons are exposed devoid of paratenon, closure of the wound with a skin flap is essential **(Figures 9.12A to G)**.

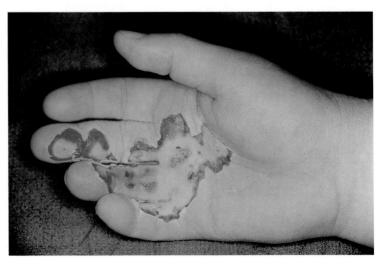

Figure 9.11A: Full thickness contact burns on the volar aspect of the hand and fingers

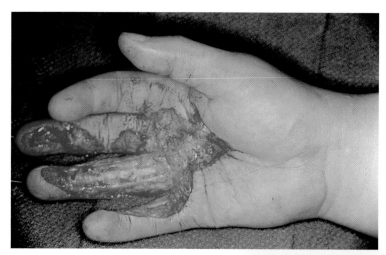

Figure 9.11B: Surgical excision of the eschar under tourniquet was performed. Note that the Paratenon on the flexor tendon of the ring finger and neurovascular bundles were preserved

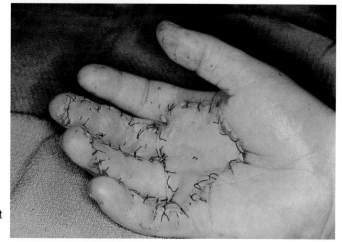

Figure 9.11C: Wound closed with thick split thickness skin grafts sutured in place

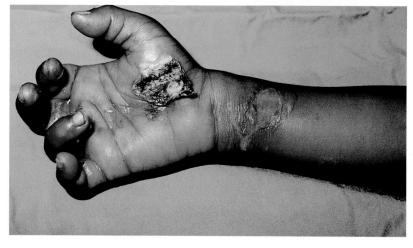

Figure 9.12A: High voltage electrical injury right hand and wrist in an 8 year old boy

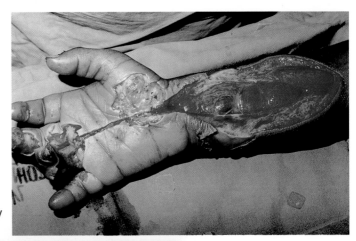

Figure 9.12B: Wounds after escharotomy and fasciotomy

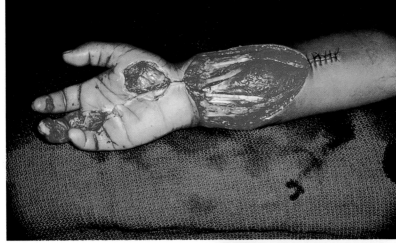

Figure 9.12C: Appearance of the wound after complete debridement and amputation of gangrenous 4th digit on 8th postburn day. Note the exposed flexor tendons at the wrist

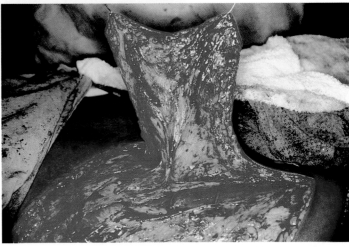

Figure 9.12D: An ipsilateral groin flap was designed and raised to cover the wrist wound

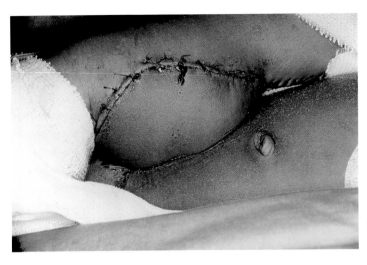

Figure 9.12E: Groin flap in place over the exposed tendon at the wrist

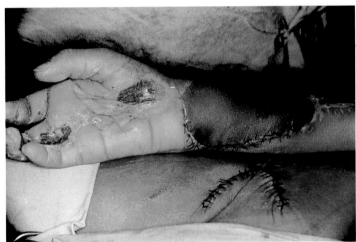

Figure 9.12F: Two weeks after surgery the groin flap was separated

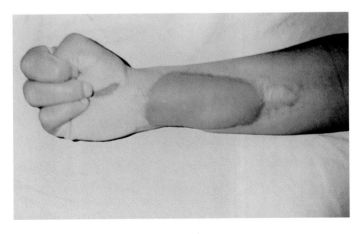

Figure 9.12G: Two years after injury, demonstrating full recovery of function

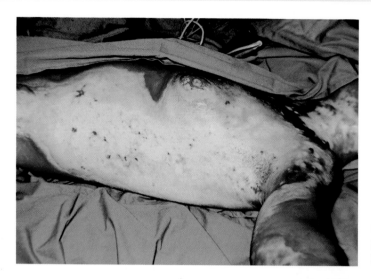

Figure 9.13A: Full thickness burns, neck, left half of the chest including the breast, abdomen and upper arm

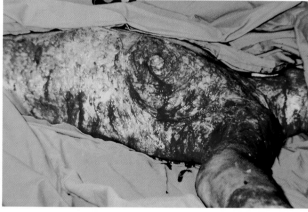

Figure 9.13B: The full thickness burns excised on the 3rd post burn day, sequentially preserving the breast volume and nipple areolar complex

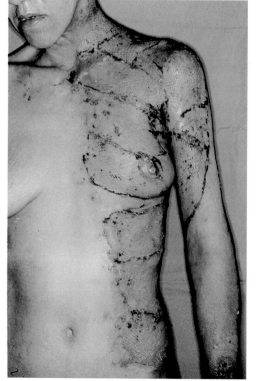

Figure 9.13C: Healed wounds 8 days after surgical excision and grafting

BURNS OF THE MAMMARY AREA

In females, burns of the chest often involve the breasts. Partial thickness burns need only the standard burn care. Deep and full thickness burns causes considerable deformity and disfigurement. Deep burns of the nipple and areolar complex having rich blood supply and epithelial source heal spontaneously.

In surgically excising burns on the chest in a female child before puberty, every effort should be taken to preserve the breast bud and nipple-areolar complex should never be excised even if it is full thickness. It may be allowed to heal even with scarring, as it forms the landmark for future reconstruction.

Full thickness burns over the breast in adult females can be excised sequentially and skin grafted, preserving the breast volume and nipple and areolar complex **(Figures 9.13A to C)**. After healing proper fitting bra should be worn to reduce contracture and hypertrophic scar formation.

BURNS OF THE PERINEUM, BUTTOCKS AND GENITALIA

Burns of the perineum are difficult to manage because of the constant soiling from bowel and bladder, that requires meticulous nursing care around the clock **(Figure 9.14)**.

A uretheral catheter should always be placed and maintained. These areas are cleaned several times a day and covered with topical antibiotic cream. Since it is difficult to apply dressings, these areas are left open. In spite of all the contamination, partial thickness burns of the perineum and upper thighs heal well.

Full thickness injuries require sequential excision and grafting. The grafts are sutured and fixed with stent tie over dressings. Preoperative bowel preparation with enemas and postoperative non-residual liquid diet for about a week must be instituted. A rectal tube is placed and sutured in place. Diversion colostomy is not necessary and should be avoided.

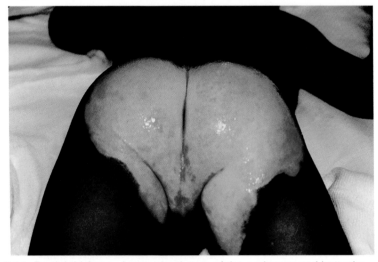

Figure 9.14: Partial thickness immersion burns of the perineum and buttocks in a 18 month boy

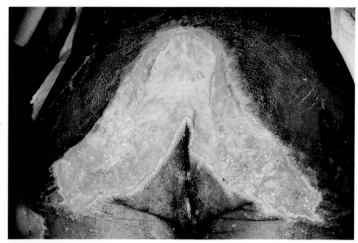

Figure 9.15A: Deep contact radiator burns on the buttocks in a 70 year old lady exposing the sacrum

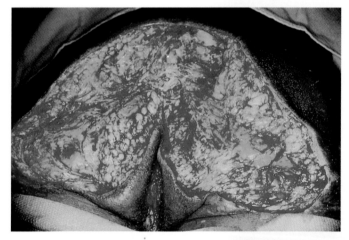

Figure 9.15B: On the 7th postburn day the wounds were excised including part of the necrotic sacrum

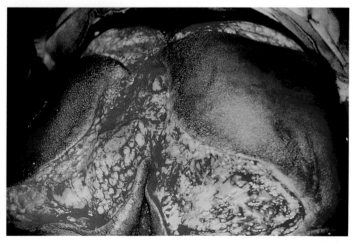

Figure 9.15C: Bilateral gluteal rotational flaps raised to close the defect

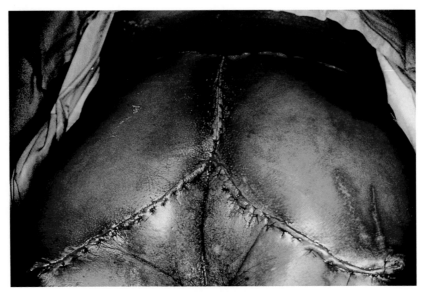

Figure 9.15D: Gluteal flaps sutured in place

Burns of the buttocks may be associated with major burns of the back of the trunk and or perineum. Because of the thick skin in this area even deep burns heal spontaneously. The constant movement of the back against the bed and dressings will have a mechanical debriding effect also.

Full thickness contact burns especially over the bony prominenses and sacrum require skin flap closure after surgical excision (Figures 9.15A to D).

Burns of the Genitalia

Burns of the genitalia in females is very rare even, with perineal burns. Burns of the penis and scrotum in males is also not very common. Most of these injuries are associated with extensive burns of the trunk and upper thighs. Isolated burn injuries in these areas are secondary to assault or abuse.

Superficial and even deep burns of the penis and scrotum heal well because of their rich blood supply. Deep burns of the scrotum may be allowed to heal as much as possible. Residual unhealed full thickness areas can be managed with excision and primary closure. In full thickness burns of the penis the deep fascia of the penis protects the deeper structures from injury. In excision of burns in this area, one should always remain above this fascia, other wise serious bleeding may be encountered. The excised areas should be covered with thick sheet skin grafts, sutured in place. Urinary catheter must be maintained at least for five days, postoperatively (Figures 9.16A to C).

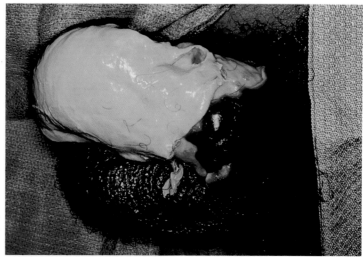

Figure 9.16A: Full thickness circumferential burns of the penis in a 42 year old male

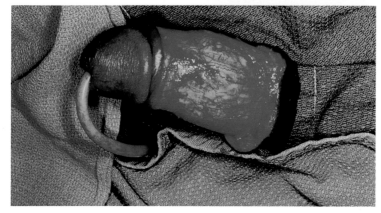

Figure 9.16B: Burn eschar excised up to the deep fascia of the penis

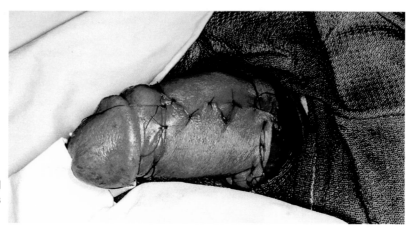

Figure 9.16C: Excised wound closed with thick sheet grafts (0.022") sutured in place

BIBLIOGRAPHY

1. Boswick JA: *The Art and Science of Burn Care.* Aspen Publication, 1987.
2. Edlich RF, Nichter JS, Morgan RF *et al:* Burns of the Head and Neck. *Otolaryngol Clin North Am* **17 (2)** : 361-88, 1984.
3. Engrav LH, Heimbach DM, Walkinshaw MD *et al:* Excison of burns of the face. *Plast Reconstr Surg* **77:**744-749, 1986.
4. Frank DH, Wachtel T, Frank HA: The early treatment and reconstruction of eyelid burns. *J Trauma* **23 (19):** 874-7, 1983.
5. Gonzalez- Ulloa M: Restoration of the face covering by means of selected skin in regional aesthetic units. *Br J Plast Surg* **9:**212-221, 1956.
6. Guy RJ, Baldwin J, Dwedar S *et al:* Three years experience in a regional burn center with burns of the eyes and eyelid. *Ophthalmic Surg* **b:**383-86, 1982.
7. Huang TT, Blackwell SJ, Lewis SR: Burn injuries of the eyelids. *Clin Plastic Surgery* **5 (4):**571-81, 1978.
8. Linhart RW: Burns of the eye and eyelids. *Ann Ophthalmology* **10(8):** 999-1001, 1998.
9. Marella Hanumadass, Richard Kagan, Takayoshi Matsuda: Early coverage of deep hand burns with groin flaps. *Journal of Trauma* **27:** 109; 1987.
10. Roger E Salisbury: Acute care of the burned hand. In Joseph G, McCarthy MD (Eds) *Plastic Surgery,* WB Saunder Company, Philadelphia **8(129):** 5399, 1990 .
11. Salisbury RE, Bevin AG: *Atlas of Reconstructive Burn Surgery,* W.B. Saunders Company 1981.
12. Wachtel TL, Frank DH. Burns of the head and neck. *Major Problems in Clinical Surgery.* W.B. Saunders company, **29:** 1984.

PART III

Management of Special Burns

10

Chemical Burns

Chemical burns are caused by contact with chemical agents that are corrosive, and in all respects is a special variety of deep burn. It can occur due to accidents in the laboratories, where corrosives are used, or in industries where they are manufactured or in homicidal burns, where corrosives are poured over the victims, particularly women. In some developing countries it is a practice to store acids for the purpose of cleaning floors and toilets. Children accidentally get access to these stored items and their curiosity will make them topple these agents on themselves. Chemical burns are seen in the modern warfare also. Adequate knowledge of this type of burns, their appearance and planning the treatment are essential.

Though the burn wound is in no way different to a thermal burn, the mechanism of progress of burn is different and treatment also is different. The primary action is to eliminate the offending agent, since the chemicals may have a prolonged action locally, as well as systemically. No delay should take place in initiating the management.

CLASSIFICATIONS OF INJURIOUS CHEMICALS

Acids, Bases, Organic Compounds and Inorganic Agents

Acids: The acids that cause burns are hydrochloric, hydrofluoric, sulfuric, nitric and phosphoric acids. Acetic acid also can cause burns.

Bases: The common bases are hydroxides of calcium, sodium, potassium and ammonia.

Organic compounds: These are the byproducts of petroleum and phenol.

Inorganic agents: Sodium sticks and chlorine gas are common examples.

Mechanism of Action

When these chemicals come into contact with the skin various kinds of reactions occur, apart from the effect of thermal burn due to the heat produced by the acid when in contact with the skin (exothermic reaction).
A. Protein denaturation occurs, resulting in corrosion of the skin.
B. Oxygen ions get into the cells and releases highly reactive chemicals and these oxidation products results in severe untoward effects on the skin.
C. These corrosives are protoplasmic poisons; they form esters with the protein and by *desiccation*, results in full thickness burn of the skin.

D. By being vesicants, they are poisonous to the proliferating cells.

E. Vesication also results in blister formation. The severity of injury depends upon:
   a. Concentration of the chemical
   b. Amount of the chemical in contact with the tissue
   c. Duration of exposure
   d. State of the lipid barrier of the skin

General Principles of Management

1. Rapid removal of all the clothing and washing with large volumes of clean cold water is very important. Any dry chemical or powder adherent to the body should be brushed away and removed before washing. Normal saline also can be used to wash the area. This procedure decreases the rate of reaction between the chemical and the tissue. This also helps the phase of the wound to become normal by the reduction of the hygroscopic action of some of the strong acids and bases. The heat that is produced in the tissues due to the reaction of the corrosive liquids with the tissues will get dissipated by this washing.

2. The treatment of chemical burns should include consideration of both local wound care and systemic support.

3. Emergency therapy consists of initial dilution, neutralization with specific concentration of solutions to prevent exothermic reactions and debridement of the burn wound, as well as facilitation of systemic detoxification and excretion of the offending agent.

4. It must be borne in mind that time should not be wasted from receiving the patient with chemical burn to initiation of treatment. The depth and magnitude of ongoing tissue necrosis is directly related to the time taken to initiate the treatment. Hence, first aid should stress on continuous irrigation of the wound with water.

5. Up to 72 hrs., the tissue necrosis will spread after contact with the chemical, till neutralization with tissue fluids take place. Hence, it is this period that has to be shortened, to reduce the damage. Patient can be even allowed to have a good shower with normal water, so that considerable dilution of the chemicals takes place.

6. As the extent of burn cannot be identified initially, fluid calculation as per normal formulae may not suffice, and these patients go into hypotension. Close monitoring of the vital signs including arterial blood gas levels; electrolytes and urinary output are necessary to predict the fluid necessary for each patient. These patients always need more fluids.

HYDROFLUORIC ACID

Hydrofluoric acid is a very strong inorganic acid, which is used in industry and in civilian life. This acid is particularly used in glass industries, by virtue of its ability to liquefy silica. It is a very lethal substance.

Clinical Presentation

Contact with the acid produces dehydration and corrosion of tissue due to free hydrogen ions, which induces skin necrosis. Cell death occurs due to the immobilization of cellular

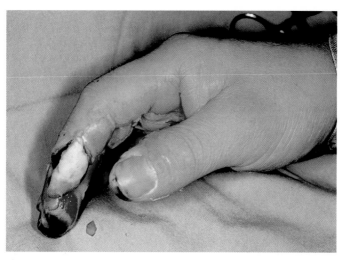

Figure 10.1: Hydrofluoric acid burns in a glass industry worker.

calcium by binding. The severity depends on the concentration, the surface area involved and the duration of exposure.

Systemic manifestation of this acid exposure comes primarily from hypocalcemia and hypomagnesemia. This induces cardiac arrhythmia such as refractory ventricular fibrillation.

Digital and hand burns are frequently seen (**Figure 10.1**). They are most painful. The skin initially appears erythematous and later, the skin assumes a gray appearance with a cheesy yellow substance beneath the skin. This progresses to full thickness burns.

Management

1. Patient with significant exposure needs to be placed in ICU with cardiac monitoring facility and pain medication is given.
2. Rapid and serial evaluation of electrolytes including calcium and magnesium are done.
3. Good IV access must be established.
4. Large doses of calcium chloride are administered intravenously.
5. ECG must be taken repeatedly.
6. Haemodialysis and induction of metabolic alkalosis are done to excrete the fluoride ions, and the serum chemistry is corrected.
7. Local treatment consists in washing the entire offending agent with lukewarm water immediately.
8. 2.5% Calcium gluconate based gel or the KY jelly are liberally applied over the area. Sometimes, calcium gluconate is injected into the subcutaneous tissues under the burnt area.
9. Some authors advocate even intra-arterial cannulation and administering calcium gluconate solution. In most instances topical application is very effective and intra-arterial injection is very much discouraged as it is associated with more complications.
10. Finally, when the general condition stabilizes, burn wounds are treated with excision and skin grafting.

Sulfuric Acid

This is a powerful descicant and has widespread use in industry. In addition to the caustic action of the acid, much heat is generated at the site of the burn which in turn produces damage. Dry hard and blackish eschars form and when they fall off, they leave behind indolent ulcers. Usually the burn occurs accidentally but is the popular acid that is thrown on the face of the victim **(Figure 10.2)** as a homicidal act or to cause disfigurement. Copious washing off the acid and supportive therapy are needed. Ulcers are often excised because they are deep and are grafted.

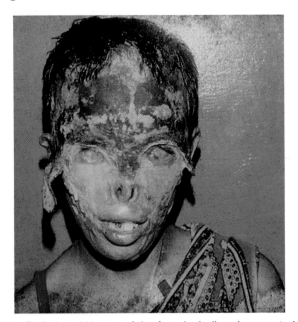

Figure 10.2: Sulfuric acid burns of the face including damage to both eyes

Hydrochloric Acid

This is a strong acid and while on contact with the skin, the burn progresses, because the acid continues to denature the protein. A coagulum forms over the affected areas under which shallow ulcers are seen. Hydrochloric acid burns are usually accidental. Treatment is excision and grafting after emergency care.

Nitric Acid

Nitric Acid is used in the jewellery industry, where it is used for polishing **(Figure 10.3)**. Both accidental burns and suicidal burns due to ingestion of the acid are common. The burnt area has a yellowish tinge. These burns are also treated with skin grafting after wound excision.

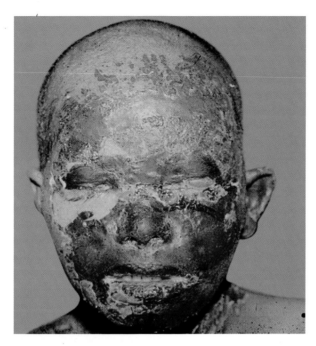

Figure 10.3: Nitric acid burns of the head and face; a homicidal attempt

Phosphorus

Commonly used in a variety of weapons of modern warfare as well as in the manufacture of crackers. While phosphorus ignites in the atmospheric air and causes burn on contact with the skin, the progress of burn goes on till the tissue is starved off oxygen. The combustion products of phosphorous are a variety of oxides and polyphosphates. Wounds are very painful and necrotic yellow eschar is seen, which has a characteristic garlic smell (Figure 10.4).

Management is to wash the area immediately with saline and saline dressings are used over the burn. Specific therapy is to irrigate with 0.5% Copper sulfate solution. This will identify the embedded phosphorus as a black film, and the agent can be removed from the area easily. Even Ultra-Violet rays are used to detect the fluorescence of phosphorus. In extensive burns, electrolyte imbalance and cardiac arrhythmias are also common. ECG monitoring is needed and ultimately grafting covers the ulcers.

BASES

These bases are proton acceptors, to which mineral alkalis belong. Alkalis catalyses protein hydrolysis. Caustic alkali burns occur with caustic soda, potassium hydroxide and lime. These cause severe burns (Figure 10.5). The exact mechanism of burn is due to extraction of water from cells, due to the hygroscopic nature of the alkali. Further the alkaline proteinates that form causes deeper tissue injury. The extent of damage depends upon the concentration, amount and condition of the skin.

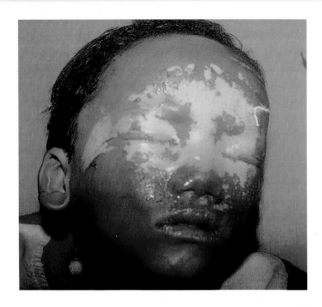

Figure 10.4: Phosphorus burns- Fire cracker injury

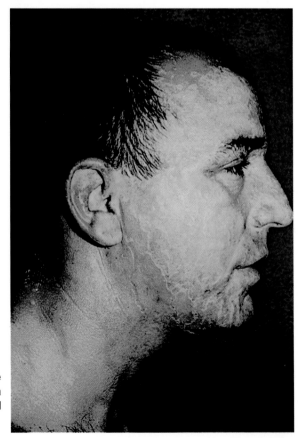

Figure 10.5: Alkali burns-"draino" a strong alkaline liquid used to clear the drain pipes was thrown on this individual's face; notice the dry, undermined and adherent Eschar in streaks

Alkali burns are penetrating burns due to saponification of dermal and sub dermal fat resulting in deep necrosis and severe pain.

Management is by washing the area affected with copious amounts of water as rapidly as possible. Washing also helps in the reduction of heat produced by the contact. The burn forms deep, desiccated and adherent eschar. These burns often require skin grafting after surgical debridement.

ORGANIC COMPOUNDS

Organic compounds will damage the cell proteins both by heat and by the direct chemical interaction with proteins, eg. phenol. The burns are like any other chemical burns. Exposure to large quantities of phenol and its absorption causes early signs of central nervous system stimulation and convulsions. Late changes include depression, respiratory failure and myocardial depression. Hypothermia due to antipyretic action mediated by hypothalamus may occur. Late complications include intravascular hemolysis, hepatic centrilobular necrosis, renal glomerular and tubular damage. Phenol should not be washed with water as dilution causes severe exothermic reaction. It should be removed with polyethylene glycol or mineral oil. The burn wounds are usually deep and require skin grafting.

INORGANIC AGENTS

Highly reactive elements like chlorine, apart from acids and alkalis causes damage to the skin directly. They directly bind with proteins, as well as producing thermal damage. Washing with liberal amounts of water and management of the thermal component of the burn are necessary. Management includes specific management and general management. General management includes: a) Critical care aspects; (b) Emergency care - Lavage with water and neutralizing agents. The latter solutions should be of the buffered variety with a pH of around 6. Strong neutralizing solutions should not be used, as further heat production may ensue in the chemical reaction (exothermic reaction). (Example: Sulfuric acid burn - neutralized with sodium hydroxide). Hence, neutralizing solutions should be used only when indicated, and that too after intensive irrigation with water.

BIBLIOGRAPHY

1. Anderson WJ, Anderson JR: Hydrofluoric acid burn of the hand, mechanism of injury and treatment. *J Hand Surgery* **13** A:52-7 ,1988.
2. Bromberg BE, Song IC, Walden RH: Hydrotherapy of chemical burns. *Plast.Recontr Surg* **35:** 85-95; 1965.
3. Curreri PW, Asch MJ, Pruitt BA: The treatment of Chemical burns. Specialized diagnostic, therapeutic and prognostic considerations. *J Trauma* **10:** 634-642, 1970.
4. Fitzpatrick KT, Moylan JA. Emergency care of chemical burns. *Postgrad Med* **78:** 189-94.
5. Herbert K, Lawrence JC. *Chemical Burns*. **15:** 381-384, 1989.
6. Herndon DN. Chemical injury. In Herndon DN (Ed). *Total Burn Care* publishers USA, **40:** 415-424.
7. Jelenko C: Chemicals that burn. *J Trauma* **14:** 65-72,1974.
8. Leonard L, Scheulen JJ, Munster A: Chemical burns- Effect of prompt first aid: *J Trauma* **22(5):**420-3, 1982.
9. Mistry D, Wainwright D: Hydrofluoric acid burns. *N Am Fam Physician* **45(4):** 1748-54; 1992.

10. Ramakrishnan, Hanumadass: *Hand Book of Burn Management*, Jaypee Bros.Medical Publishers, **17**:152-159;1989.
11. Sawhney CP, Koushikh R. Acid and alkali burns: considerations in their management. *Burns* **15**: 132-35; 1989.
12. Terry H. Caustic soda burns: their prevention and treatment. *Br Med J* **1**:756, 1943.

11

Electrical Burns

After the development of the electric lamp by Thomas Edison, electricity has made significant impact on human civilization. Since the first report of death from electrical injury in 1879, several clinical and experimental reports on various aspects of electrical trauma have appeared in the literature. Despite an increased awareness of the potential dangers, electricity is responsible for many fatalities all over the world. Although, high-voltage (>1,000volts) electrical trauma accounts for a small portion of all electrical injuries, it is, nevertheless, responsible for devastating injuries affecting multiple organ system. In recent years, significant advancement has been made in the management of electrical injuries due to better understanding of pathophysiology and multidisciplinary approach of treatment resulting in a low mortality. Surgical management of electrical trauma continues to be a major challenge. It is still responsible for very high number of major limb amputations resulting in lifelong disability in young individuals.

Major electrical *Burns* constitute approximately three percent of all admissions to major burn centers. About 1,000 electrical deaths occur annually in the United States, 200 of them in lineman or other employees of utility companies. Approximately one third of high voltage injuries occur in electrical workers, and one-third in construction workers and the remainder results from non-work or home accidents. With increasing production of electrical energy to meet the demands of our technological age, the frequency of electrical injuries has significantly increased. An understanding of the mechanism involved is basic to intelligent care of patients surviving the initial insult.

Electrical injuries, unlike thermal burns, often cause massive tissue damage underneath intact skin. Exposure of this tissue damage uncovers vital structures such as nerves, tendons, and joints, which then require coverage. These injuries remain a diagnostic and therapeutic challenge during the acute post-injury period, but even after recovery, these patients may develop long-term problems such as neuropathies, cataracts and atypical pain syndromes.

TERMS AND TECHNICAL ASPECTS OF ELECTRICAL INJURIES

The effect and degree of damage inflicted upon the human body by electricity is dependant upon the type of current, amperage, voltage, resistance at the point of contact, path the current takes through the body, the duration of contact, individual susceptibility, and other variable factors such as the humidity of the air, and the size, and nature of the electrodes.

Type of Current

In general alternating current is more dangerous than direct current of similar intensity. The alternations cause tetanic spasms which make the victim grip the electrodes more firmly and increase the difficulty of detachment, thereby augmenting the insult which is proportionate to the duration of flow of current through the body.

Amperage

The degree of tissue damage in a given electrical injury is proportional to the intensity of current (amperage) which flows through the tissue as stated in Ohm's law:

$$\text{Amperage (intensity)} = \frac{\text{Voltage (tension or potential)}}{\text{Resistance}}$$

Ohm's equation indicates that higher the electrical potential the greater is the intensity of the current; likewise decreasing the resistance in the tissue results in increased intensity of current.

Voltage

Electrical current less than 1,000 volts is considered low-tension current and above 1,000 volts, high-tension current. High-tension wires usually carry alternating current of higher voltage and amperage. Voltages over 40 volts should be considered dangerous. Low voltage alternating current can readily induce cardiac arrhythmia and death under the proper circumstances.

The risk of thermal injuries is proportional to the voltage. Extensive *Burns* after high-tension accidents are partly caused by arcing of the current, which consists of ionized air particles, and much of the electrical energy is then consumed resulting in considerable voltage drop.

Resistance

The resistance of the body tissues to the flow of a current, in order of decreasing magnitude is: bone, fat, tendon, skin, muscle, blood, and nerve. The skin resistance, being the most important, varies within wide limits depending upon its thickness, moisture and cleanliness. The resistance offered by the calloused palm and sole may reach one million ohms, while the average normal skin resistance is 1,000 ohms. If the cutaneous resistance is low at the site of current entrance, systemic damage may be greater; conversely if the skin resistance remains high, local damage is more severe and systemic injury is minimized. After an electric current has penetrated the skin, it passes rapidly through the paths of least resistance through body fluids and along blood vessels and nerves before it collects again at the points of exit (grounding) from the body.

The combination of high internal resistance and comparatively small cross-section of the limb causes a considerable voltage drop when the current flows through. The resulting transformation of electrical energy into heat is maximal at the contact site, thus affecting the skin and the adjacent tissues. As the tissue resistance of the trunk is lower and its cross-sectional area much greater, the amount of heat released is considerably less, and thermal damage to internal organs is therefore rare.

Path of the Current

Once the flow of current is established through the victim, the path followed by the current is variable and determines both the immediate and later effects of injury.

The most severe local lesions, which also has a higher incidence of complications, are found in the pathway of greatest resistance, i.e., from hand to hand, or from hand to foot, while current flow through the lowest resistance pathway - in and out of the same extremity - causing less serious damage. If the heart or brain stem has been traversed, respiratory paralysis is more frequent in injuries due to high voltage alternating currents.

Low and High-tension Injuries

In the low-tension group the victim often gets locked to the contact and occurs most frequently when the current went in and out of the same extremity. The most characteristic lesion encountered in this group is a small deep burn, which sometimes deep enough to involve vessels, tendons, and nerves. A common feature of low-tension contact *Burns* are their localization to the hands or to the mouth. The typical electrical *Burns* of the lips represent an exception to the rule that the severity of the lesion depends on the resistance of the current pathway. The current circuit is short, and the resistance of the richly vascularized tissue is small.

In the high-tension accidents, locking to the contact is not common. The persons are thrown away from the contact and thus acquire fractures, brain hemorrhages, rupture of the spleen, and other severe injuries. The infrequency of locking with higher voltages is probably explained by the fact that the circuit is completed by arcing before the person touches the contact. In this group, systemic effects on the central nervous system are most characteristic.

Location of the Burn

The points of contact (Entrance) and grounding (Exit) in many cases are difficult to determine because of extensive associated arc and flame *Burns* that obscure the contact and exit points. *Burns* of the arms and hands are most common followed by *Burns* of the legs and feet, scalp, and trunk.

The resistance of the cranial bones is probably mainly due to the outer and inner tables, as the highly vascular layer of diploe is supposed to be a good conductor. The large voltage drop in the skin, galea, and outer table results in the heat being largely dissipated on the outside, thus sparing the brain from direct thermal injury.

Although the rate of current flow through the trunk is generally insufficient to cause injury to internal organs, the heart may suffer fatal disturbance of the pacemaker mechanism, and sudden death at the time of the accident may result from ventricular fibrillation. Ventilatory assistance and external cardiac massage may therefore be of great value immediately following injury.

PATHOLOGY

The principal pathologic change caused by electricity is coagulation necrosis. In contrast to thermal burn, electrical injury is classically deep and accompanied by muscle damage. Vascular lesions dominate the clinical picture in many electrical injuries. Arterial changes in the vicinity of electrical *Burns* are due to the heat rather than the specific action of the electrical current. Thrombi are apt to form within the damaged vessels and ischemic necrosis is therefore common in high-tension injuries. Narrowing of the arteries persistent 3 months after the injury is probably due to scar formation in and around the vessel wall, with consequent decrease in blood flow.

Permanent changes in peripheral nerves usually do not extend beyond the area of local destruction. Functional changes occur mainly in motor fibers and are rapidly reversible.

Recent Theories on the Pathogenesis of Tissue Damage

To understand the effect of electrical forces on biological systems, it is helpful to think in terms of bioelectrical circuits. The major portion of cellular energy, for example is expended in maintaining the difference in electrolyte concentrations (and secondary transmembrane potentials) across cell membranes. Ions leak across membranes by electrodifusion and are pumped back in by ATP-driven pumps. The vital cell membrane property which limits this leakage is resistance to ion transport, which in turn serves to conserve energy.

Strong electric fields in tissues cause lethal cellular damage by at least three mechanisms: Joule's heating, electroporation and electroconformational alteration of membrane proteins. These mechanisms cause increased membrane permeability and lead to energy depletion. In Joule's heating, the passage of electrical current through conducting material causes its temperature to rise. The lipid bilayer of the cell membrane is perhaps the most heat-sensitive structure in the cell. Disruption of cell membrane occurs at temperatures greater than 42°C. At slightly higher temperatures (>45°C), disruption of intramolecular bonds in proteins, with loss of conformation (denaturation), takes place. At temperatures above 65° C, DNA denatures. Heat damage is also related to duration of exposure. The higher the temperature, the shorter the exposure time required for adverse effects. In most cases of high-voltage electrical shock (1-to-10 KV), heat damage occurs instantaneously at skin contact points but computational simulations suggest that current passage for 1-3 seconds is required to thermally burn tissues between contact points. The susceptibility to heat damage is quite similar for all mammalian cells. Another recognized mechanism of electrical trauma is electroporation, the process of structural breakdown of membranes by strong electric fields, which was first identified in the mid-1980's. The normal transmembrane potential for mammalian cell is less than 0.1 volts. During electrical shock, electrical current flowing around the cell causes supraphysiologic transmembrane potential to be established across the membranes of very large cells. Skeletal muscle and nerve cells are much larger than other cells, experience this effect most severely. When the transmembrane potential exceeds 8-10 times normal (~ 1 volt), the membrane swells with water until it ruptures. This process is called electroporation and it can happen quickly, in less than 1 millisecond. Tissue field-strengths in the 100 volt/cm range can electroporate skeletal muscle and peripheral nerve cells, whereas field are 1000 times larger are required to electroporate fibroblasts and endothelial or other smaller cells. During electrical shock, fields in the tissue can be expected to range between 1 to 1,000 volts/cm.

The pattern of tissue injury manifested is also a consequence of the body's electrical properties. All tissues except the epidermis are relatively good conductors. When a victim comes into contact with a power source (> 200 volts), the epidermis is usually destroyed by heat within milliseconds. Large currents can then pass and produce tissue damage, particularly to skeletal muscle and nerve.

Recently, another type of injury mechanism has been proposed; electroconformational denaturation of membrane proteins, particularly ion channels. When the transmembrane potential exceeds 0.6 to 0.8 volts, the potassium channel is damaged, and this leads to cell dysfunction. Other channels have higher thresholds.

Disruption of membrane integrity by heat, electroporation, or electroconformational protein damage leads to osmotic swelling of tissues. Alternately, this can precipitate, as it commonly does, muscle compartment syndromes. When muscle compartment pressures exceed 30-35 cm of water, the vascular circulation is compromised, and this can cause ischemic necrosis.

Fasciotomies to relieve this pressure must be completed in 4 to 6 hours to prevent ischemic necrosis of the muscle. Unless there has been significant heating, however, the damaged tissue appears grossly normal immediately after injury. Typically, it is at least 1 to 3 days before the true extent of damage becomes clear. The problem is compounded by the fact that healthy skin and fat often conceal injured muscle, nerve, and bone. Thus, a major problem is the difficulty of accurately diagnosing and localizing tissue damage scattered throughout the current path before cellular degeneration occurs.

TYPES OF INJURY

The typical types of tissue destruction resulting from electrical injury are: Entry and exit wounds, (Contact and grounding points) arc *Burns* (or "markings"), and thermal burns. *Entry and exit Wounds*: The term entry and exit wound is a misnomer as the alternating current does not exit. However, in direct high voltage electrical injury or true electrical injury, these terms have been used for a longtime and are popular, indicating the contact and grounding points. A true high-tension electrical injury has the classic clinical features of a well demarcated leathery full thickness site of current entrance (contact) and exit (grounding). Although, the distinction between entrance and exit wound is not always obvious.

Entrance and Exit Wounds

The typical entry wound is charred and depressed and blisters may be produced by vaporization of water within the tissues (Figure 11.1). Circumscribed zone of tissue coagulation necrosis is seen at the exit (grounding) point (Figure 11.2). Various degrees of tissue damage can be assumed to lie in the deeper tissues adjacent to the points of current entrance and exit. The extensive underlying tissue damage is suspected by the intense and immediate swelling extending from the entry wound. When the body becomes the conduit for electrical current

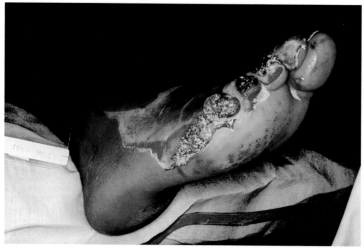

Figure 11.1: Typical contact point or entry wound; charred, depressed and diffuse in nature

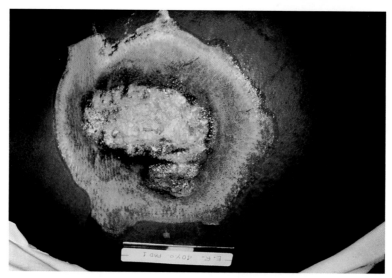

Figure 11.2: Typical grounding point, or exit wound; circumscribed zone of coagulation necrosis

to ground, the injuries produced result from the conversion of electrical to heat energy. The resultant damage is a function of the resistance of individual tissues and their sensitivity to heat damage. In general, the higher the resistance of the tissue at the point of contact and the higher the voltage, the deeper and more extensive the tissue damage. Bone has the greatest resistance to current flow and therefore generates the most heat, but bone structure makes it most resistance to heat damage. Nerves and blood vessels which most readily transmit current, generate only a small amount of heat, but are the most sensitive to heat damage **(Figures 11.3 and 11.4).**

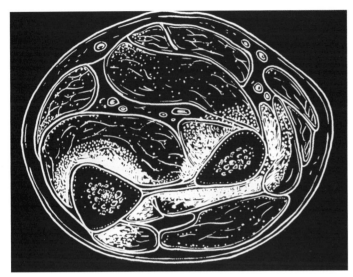

Figure 11.3: Diagram showing periosseous necrosis of muscle and soft tissue with viable superficial muscles and skin (Reproduced with kind permission from WB Saunders Company: Hal Bingham, MD Chapter on Electrical Burns in "Clinics in Plastic Surgery—Advances in Burn Care." January 1986, Volume 13, No. 1. Page 78, Figure 4))

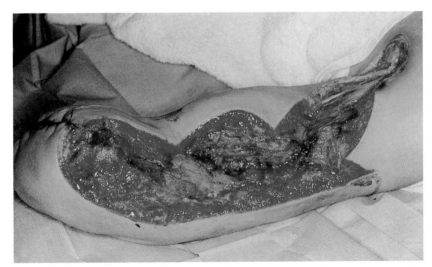

Figure 11.4: High voltage electrical injury, of the upper extremity with necrosis of deep muscles around the humerus; whereas the superficial muscles and soft tissue are intact

The flow of current from the entry point usually along the path of least resistance, indicating one or more tracts of damage. At the grounding point, the energy collects again producing an extensive core of tissue necrosis.

Arc Burn

Electrical injury produced by current coursing external to the body from the contact point to ground is called Arc Burn. The heat generated by the arcing *Burns* is often in the range of

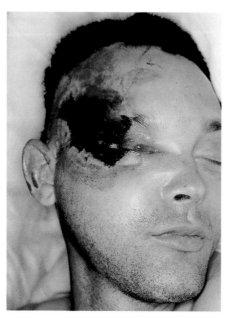

Figure 11.5: Arc burn sustained in a suicidal attempt; fell on the third rail of a railway track

3,000 to 20,000 degrees centigrade and the depth of these *Burns* is dependent upon the proximity of the current to the skin. Extremely high voltage (50,000 volts or more) may result in a burn which covers all the body suface exposed to the heat. These are uncommon and tend to give localized deep *Burns* **(Figure 11.5)**.

Electrical Flame Burns

Thermal *Burns* result from instantaneous ignition of clothing or environmental object by the current. These *Burns* have the characteristics of the usual thermal *Burns* but are usually full thickness injury owing to long exposure of the dazed or unconscious patient to the flame.

WOUND MANAGEMENT

The management of electrical *Burns* has been a subject of considerable controversy. Opinions varying on immediate excision, delayed complete debridement and allowing wounds to separate by sloughing of dead tissue. The dilemma is simplified if the time of surgical debridement is individualized according to the extensiveness of tissue destruction, the type of injury (entry and exit, arc, or flame).

Fasciotomy

Compartment syndromes are a dreaded complication of electrical *Burns* of the extremities. These injuries require frequent evaluation of all extremities with particular attention paid to the development of swelling, deep pain, and paresthesias. The presence or absence of pulses is an extremely poor indicator of increasing compartment pressures. While careful monitoring of compartment pressure may be performed using a variety of catheter techniques, aggressive fasciotomy of affected tissues in the operating room is the treatment of choice for preventing progressive tissue ischemia.

Fasciotomy has both therapeutic and diagnostic role in electrical injuries. Indications are cyanosis of the distal uninjured skin, impaired capillary filling in the nail beds, progressive neurologic changes, and brawny edema with extreme tightness of muscle compartments on palpation. The confinement of swelling in damaged muscle by the fascial investment of the individual muscle compartments may prevent adequate distal flow even though the overlying skin is not sufficiently taut to indicate the need for fasciotomy.

It may be necessary to determine the site and extent of necrotic muscle masses, because if undetected they result in early toxicity (within 3-5 days) results in liquefaction, and infected abscess produce concealed lethal sepsis. The danger of sepsis following fasciotomy is reduced by topical antibiotics. Adequate fasciotomy consist of an incision through the skin and subcutaneous tissue and incision of the investing fascia of all muscle compartments. Adequate fasciotomy however, does not always assure survival of muscle masses.

Tetanus Immunization and Antibiotics

Tetanus prophylaxis should be administered initially and is important because of the depth of the electrical injury. Penicillin is administered parenterally for 10 days or until it is certain that all necrotic muscle has been removed by debridement as a prophylaxis against clostridial infections.

Amputations

There is no necessity to perform emergency amputations in most cases. If the patient develops intractable metabolic acidosis and/or pigments in the urine not clearing with fluids and diuretics, one should consider medical amputations by application of a rubber tornique around the damaged limb and freezing it with dry ice (Figure 11.6). In general, necessary amputations can most safely be accomplished on the second or third day post-injury after patient is fully stabilized and is a better candidate for general anesthesia. Indications for amputation are, massive circumferential devitalized muscle with gross evidence of gangrene, carbonization, and ' for surgical revision of autoamputation by electric current (Figures 11.7A and 11.7B). The initial use of fasciotomy often defines the extent of debridement or level of amputation which will ensure the least number of complications and the best chance for survival. Amputations within a few hours of injury is reserved as mentioned before for those few patients whose response to shock therapy is unsatisfactory. The most common problem with early amputation is the exposure of large areas which are of questionable viability.

Entry and Exit Wounds

The most controversial issue in wound management is the optimal time for excision of limited areas of tissue necrosis associated with entry or exit wounds, or small deep arc burns. These wounds are treated initially with topical chemotherapy. Once the resuscitation is completed

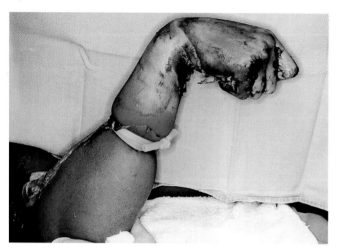

Figure 11.6: Medical amputation of the hand and forearm by application of a tornique proximal to the gangrene and freezing the limb with dry ice

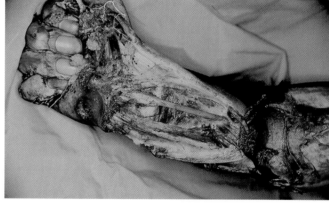

Figure 11.7A: Thirty two year old man was under the influence of alcohol when he climbed an electrical pole and touched a cable carrying 7,200 volts. The right upper extremity, the site of entrance was totally gangrenous

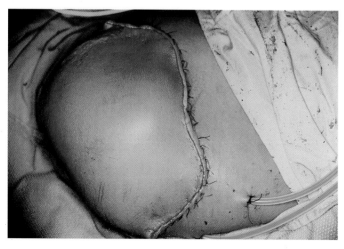

Figure 11.7B: On the third post-burn day, a right glenohumeral disarticulation was performed

and the patient is stable, debridement of the nonviable tissue should be done within 48 hours. At this time, definitive closure of the wounds including amputation stumps should not be contemplated. The open wounds should be covered with cadaver homografts or other biological or antimicrobial dressing. A second look procedure under anesthesia in the operation room may be indicated in extensive deep injury on 4 or 5th day. One should wait at least 8 to 10 days before definitive wound closure. An exception to this rule is in special areas like scalp injuries with exposed skull, where one can excise the scalp wound and cover the devitalized skull with an immediate local flap.

Definitive wound closure should be attempted after complete debridement of all non-viable tissue has been achieved and no further progression of necrosis is observed. In the majority of cases, autografts and secondary closure of amputation stumps may be sufficient. In cases, where vital structures are exposed, flap coverage may be necessary **(Figures 11.8 A to F)**. The general plan of management of wound is altered if local or systemic signs of infection or toxicity supervene. Septic complications most often arise from hidden extensive deep tissue

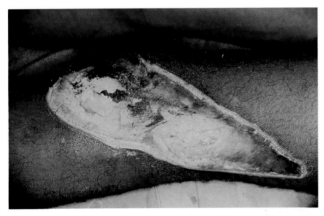

Figure 11.8A: An exit wound on the lateral aspect of the knee in the patient illustrated in Figure 11.7

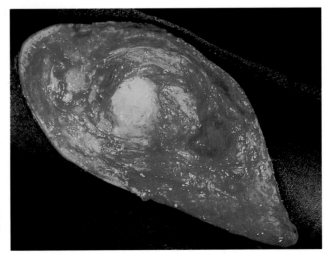

Figure 11.8B: Wound after debridement and excision of the necrotic lateral condyles of the femur and tibia

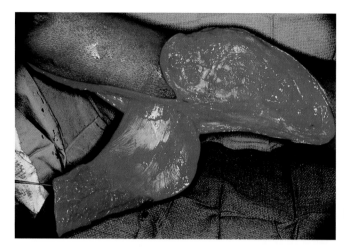

Figure 11.8C: A gastrocnemius muscle flap was raised

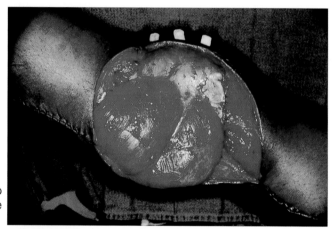

Figure 11.8D: The muscle flap was utilized to cover the lateral aspect of the exposed knee joint and bones

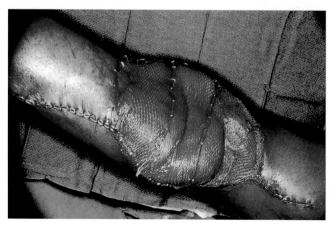

Figure 11.8E: Muscle flap was covered with split thickness skingrafts

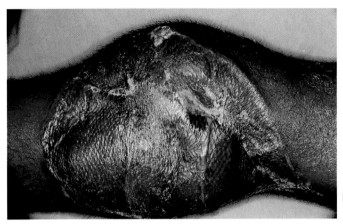

Figure 11.8F: Healed wounds two weeks after flap closure

necrosis which was overlooked in the initial evaluation. Sepsis is often first detected by mild disorientation and tachycardia. Immediate surgical exploration of all wounds is carried out when sepsis which cannot be attributed to other frequent causes in burn patients supervenes burn wound sepsis such as, pulmonary complications or indwelling venous catheter sepsis. The location of entry and exit wounds often presents special problems of wound management. Immediate exploration is necessary when the abdominal contents are damaged by a through and through abdominal wall injury. If the location of the wound is situated directly over a major blood vessel or nerve it is best treated by early exploration, adequate debridement and closure with a full thickness pedicle graft or a sliding graft.

Arc Burn

They vary in extent and depth. The deep second or third degree wounds involving extensive skin surfaces are managed as ordinary thermal burns. The charred, depressed, localized arc wound is unusually deep and often extends through all layers of tissue to involve muscle, tendon, and neurovascular bundles. These wounds are treated like the entry and exit wounds.

Cutaneous and Thermal Burns

These *Burns* result from the heat generated from the arc-ing spray of intense heat generated (4,000 to 20,000 degrees centigrade) or from flame *Burns* ignited by electricity. These injuries are treated like any other flame *Burns* with early excision and split thickness skin grafting.

REGIONAL ELECTRICAL BURN WOUND MANAGEMENT

Scalp and Skull

Electrical injuries of the scalp and cranium are usually the result of contact with a high tension source, the feet or hands functioning as for grounding or point of exit. The extent of irreversible soft tissue damage may not be immediately apparent. The treatment of an electrical injury has been based on the depth of tissue loss. With loss of pericranium and exposure or involvement of the underlying bone, the approach in the past, frequently has been conservative.

If the periosteum is lost, sequestration occurs over many months. In skull injuries, removal of the outer table and coverage of the bleeding surface with a split-thickness skin graft will speed healing (See chapter on the management of burn wounds in special areas).

With involvement and loss of the entire thickness of the skull, one hopes for an intact dura. Delay, while awaiting sequestration, often is complicated by the occurrence of epidural abscesses or meningitis. On the other hand, early excision of bone invites the possible complications of hemorrhage, CSF leaks, and meningitis. If the injury is full thickness and the diploic cavity is destroyed, then the third option is early excision of the eschar and definitive flap coverage of the underlying exposed bone. Such an approach regards the devitalized bone as an in situ bone graft that will prosper beneath well-vascularized tissue. If debridment and definitive coverage can be obtained before the bone becomes osteomyelitic, this approach is uniformly successful. (See chapter on the management of burn wounds in special areas). If the coverage defect is sufficiently large that the remaining uninjured scalp is inadequate to cover the exposed bone, free microvascular transfer of muscle or perhaps omentum is indicated.

Mouth, Lips and Tongue

Electrical *Burns* of the mouth are infrequent injuries but are the most common types of electrical trauma in children. Most such *Burns* are caused by a multiple-outlet extension cords. The child sucks an open outlet and completes the circuit. The mechanism of injury is probably a combination of an electric arc or flash burn, and contact burn. Most of these wounds are more extensive than they first appear; the extent of injury becomes apparent only after several days **(Figures 11.9 to 11.11)**. Children with perioral electrical *Burns* should

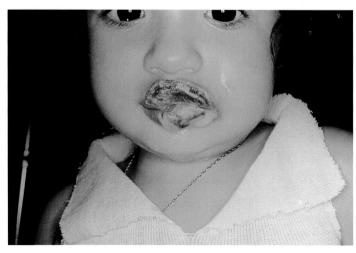

Figure 11.9: Electrical burns of the both upper and lower lips in a 18 month old child

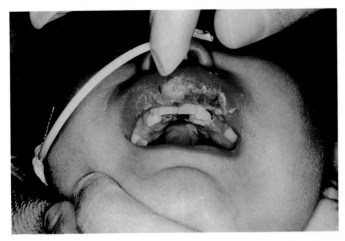

Figure 11.10: Electrical burns of the upper lip with involvement of the hard palate

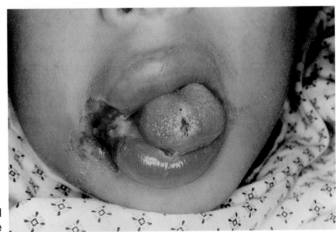

Figure 11.11: Electrical burns of the oral commissure with involvement of the tongue

be hospitalized and observed for possible systemic effects of electrical injury, as well as feeding difficulties and bleeding episodes. Tetanus immunization has to be updated in all cases. Prophylactic antibiotics usually are not necessary.

Children who develop feeding difficulties because of drooling, secondary to swelling and associated intraoral injury may be fed entirely with a nasogastric tube. The wounds can be managed conservatively by cleaning them periodically with hydrogen peroxide. Secondary hemorrhage may occur from labial artery. Wounds are allowed to heal by secondary intention. After complete healing the patients should be fitted with microstomia prevention splints. These children should be observed for 6 months to a year, for the development of any defects. Surgical corrections must be instituted promptly for established deformities.

Hands

No area of the body has stimulated as much controversy as electrical *Burns* of the hand, as this part of the body is more frequently injured than other areas because of its unique functional

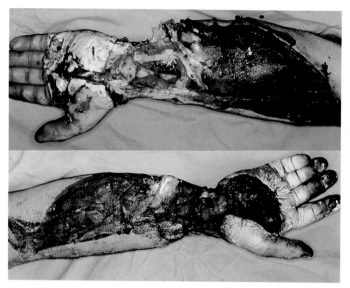

Figure 11.12A: A twenty six year old man was installing a T.V. antenna, when he slipped and came in contact with an electrical power line carrying 10,000 volts. The entrance wounds are on both hands and wrists. Both hands are gangrenous with circumferential necrosis of all the muscles of the distal forearms

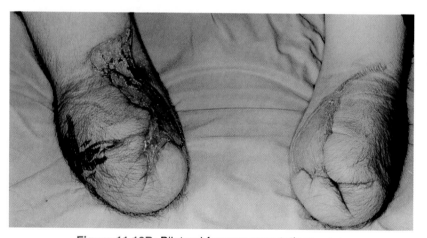

Figure 11.12B: Bilateral forearm amputations were performed one week after the injury

ability. Electrical current which enters the volar surface of the hand causes spasm of the finger flexors, uniting the patient to the electrical source and resulting in severe *Burns* **(Figures 11.12A and B)**. Nerve damage is most often encountered. In the primary treatment of *Burns* of the hands, excellent results are obtained by primary surgical excision and secondary closure of the wound, either by skin grafting or flap closure (See chapter on the management of burn wounds in special areas).

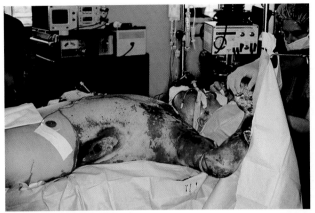

Figure 11.13A: A 22-year-old construction worker came in contact with electrical transmission lines carrying 20,000 volts. The entrance wound is on left upper extremity, the exit wound is on the left flank extending deep to the transverses abdominal muscle

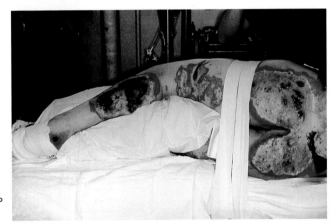

Figure 11.13B: Patient also sustained 52% full thickness flash and arc burns

Trunk

Primary excision of burned tissues is indicated in selected cases **(Figures 11.13A to D)**. Intra-abdominal lesions following electrical injuries which include necrosis of the gallbladder, perforation of a hallow viscera, pancreatitis, transient ileus, Curling's ulcer has been reported. Renal injury with acute tubular necrosis and uremia has contributed to several fatalities of surviving victims of initial electrical insult **(Figure 11.14A to D)**.

SEQUELAE

The residual effects of electrical injury are frequent, often not apparent for months, and occur in organs or areas not presenting abnormal findings during the acute course of the illness. The long interval between injury and the appearance of tissue damage is similar in time to the effects of radiation. Common sequelae are most frequently observed in the eye (cataract), neurologic function (quadriplegia, paraplegia, causalgia, convulsions, and headache) and gastrointestinal tract (cholelithiasis), and bone sequestra.

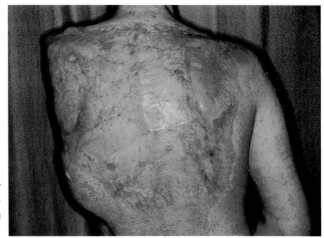

Figure 11.13C: Patient, 8 weeks after injury and after undergoing left shoulder disarticulation, debridement of the exit wound, excision of full thickness burns and autografting

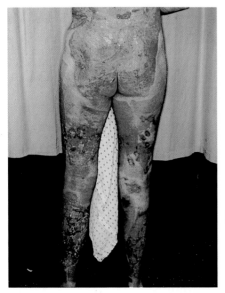

Figure 11.13D: Multiple excisions and homografting and auto grafting was done to close all the wound

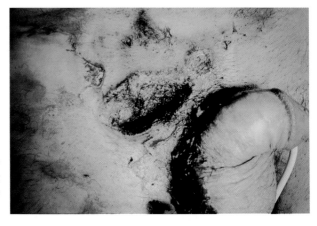

Figure 11.14A: The exit wound on the lower abdomen and the inguinal area destroying the right spermatic cord, in the same patient illustrated in the Figure 11.12

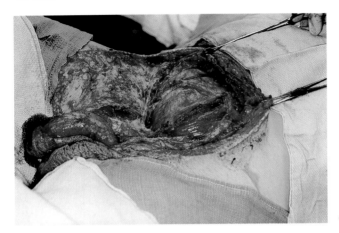

Figure 11.14B: Appearance of the wound after complete debridement on the 7th post-burn day

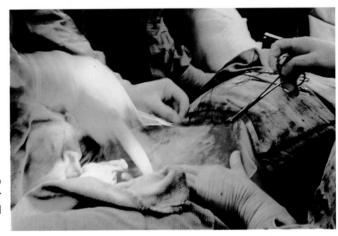

Figure 11.14C: Marlex mesh was used to repair the abdominal wall. Ten days later granulation tissue grew through the mesh and the wound was covered with autografts

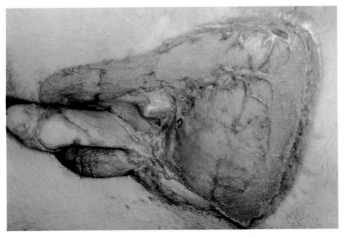

Figure 11.14D: Completely healed wound 3 months after injury

BIBLIOGRAPHY

1. Achauer B, Applebaum R, Vander KVM: Electrical burn injury to upper extremity. *Br J Plast Surg* **47**:331, 1994.
2. Artz CP: Changing concept of electrical injury. *Am J Surg* 128: 600, 1974.
3. Baxter CR: Present concepts in the management of major electrical injury. *Surg Clin North Am* **50**: 1401, 1970.
4. Bingham H: Electrical burns. *Clin Plast Surg* **13**: 75, 1986.
5. Boggid H, Freund L Bagger JP: Persistent atrial fibrillation following electrical injury. *Occupational Medicine* 45: 49-50,1995.
6. Butler ED and Gant TD: Electrical injuries, with special reference to the upper extremities. *Am J Surg* **134:** 95, 1977.
7. Bywater EGL, Beall D: Crush injuries with impairment of renal function. *BMJ* **1:** 427-32, 1941.
8. Chandra NC, Siu CO, Munster AM: Clinical predictors of myocardial damage after high-voltage electrical injury. *Crit Care Med* 18:293-7,1990.
9. Chen CT, Aarsvold JN, Block TA, *et al:* Radionuclide probes for tissue damage. *Ann NY Acad Sci* **720:** 181-91, 1994.
10. Cravalho EG, Toner M, Gaylor D, *et al:* Response of cells to supraphysiologic temperatures: experimental measurements and kinetic models. In: Lee RC, Cravalho EG, Burke JF (Eds) *Electrical Trauma: The Pathophysiology, Manifestations, and Clinical Management.* Cambridge: Cambridge University press, 281-300,1992.
11. d'Amato TA, Kaplan IB, Britt LD: High-voltage electrical injury: A role for mandatory exploration of deep muscle compartments. *J Natl Med Assoc* **86:** 535, 1994.
12. Daniel RK, Ballard PA, Heroux P, *et al:* High-voltage electrical injury. *J Hand Surg [Am]* **13:** 44-9, 1988.
13. Diller KR: The mechanisms and kinetics of heat injury accumulation. *Ann NY Acad Sci* **720:** 38-55, 1994.
14. DiVincenti FC, Moncrief JA, and Pruitt BA: Electrical injuries: A review of 65 cases. *J Trauma* **9:** 497-507,1969.
15. Esses SI and Peters WJ: Electrical burns; pathophysiology and complications. *Can J Surg* **24:** 11,1981.
16. Fish R: Electric Shock, Part I: Nature and Mechanism of injury. *J Emerg Med* **11:** 309-312, 1993.
17. Fish R: Electric Shock, Part II: Nature and Mechanism of injury. *J Emerg Med* **11:** 457-462, 1993.
18. Haberal MA: An eleven-year survey of electrical burn injuries. *J Burn Care Rehabil* **16:** 43-48, 1995.
19. Hanumadass ML, Voora SB, Kagan RJ and Matsuda T: Acute electrical burns: a 10 -year clinical experience. *Burns* 12:427-31, 1986.
20. Himel HN, Ahn LC, Jones KC, *et al:* Scavenging high-voltage wire, a hazardous petty larceny. *J Emerg Med* 10:285-9,1992.
21. Holliman CJ, Saffle JR, Kravitz M, *et al:* Early surgical decompression in the management of electrical injuries. *Am J Surg* **144:** 733,1982.
22. Hunt JL, Sato RM and Baxter: Acute electrical *Burns* current diagnostic and therapeutic approaches to management. *Arch Surg* **115:** 434, 1980.
23. Hussmann J, Kucan JO, Russell RC, *et al:* Electrical injuries-morbidity, outcome and treatment rationale. *Burns* 21:530-535, 1995.
24. Ku CS, In SL, Hsu XL, *et al:* Myocardial damage associated with electrical injury. *Am Heart J* **118:** 621-4,1989.
25. Lee RC, Gaylor DG, Bhatt DL, *et al:* Role of cell membrane rupture in the pathogenesis of electrical trauma. *J Surg Res* **44:** 709-19,1988.
26. Lee RC, Kolodney MS: Electrical injury mechanisms: electrical breakdown of cell membranes. *Plast Reconstr Surg* **80:** 672-79,1987.
27. Lee RC: Injury by Electrical Forces: Pathophysiology, Manifestations, and Therapy. *Curr Probl Surg* **34(9):** 677-765, 1997.
28. Levine NS, Atkins A, McKeel DW Jr, *et al:* Spinal cord injuries following electrical accidents: case report. *J Trauma* **15:** 459-63, 1975.

29. Luce EA and Gottlieb SE: 'True' high-tension electrical injuries. *Ann Plast Surg* **12:** 321-325, 1984.
30. Luce EA: The spectrum of electrical injuries. In: Lee RC, Cravalho EG, Burke IF (Eds). Electrical trauma. New York: Cambridge University press, 106, 1993.
31. Mann R, Gibran N, Engrav L, *et al:* Is immediate decompression of high voltage electrical injuries to the upper extremity always necessary? *J Trauma* **40:** 584-589, 1996.
32. Mann RJ and Wallquist JM: Early decompression fasciotomy in the treatment of high-voltage electrical *Burns* of extremities. *South Med J* **68:** 1103, 1975.
33. Moran KT, Thupari JN, Munster AM: Electrical and lightning induced cardiac arrest reversed by prompt cardiopulmonary resuscitation [letter] *JAMA* **255:** 211-57, 1986.
34. Nafs F, Aromir F, Carreira S, *et al:* High-tension electrical burns. A review of 85 patients. *Eur J Plast Surg* **16:** 84, 1993.
35. National Safety Council: Accident Facts: 1983. Chicago: National safety council; 1983.
36. Parshley P, Kilgore J, Pulito J, *et al:* Aggressive approach to the extremity damaged by electric current. *Am J Surgl* **50:** 78, 1985.
37. Petty PG, Parkin G: Electrical injury to the central nervous system. *Neurosurgery* **19:** 282-5, 1986.
38. Powell KT, Morgenthaler AW, Weaver JC: Tissue electroporation: observation of reversible breakdown in viable frog skin. *Biophys J* **56:** 1163-71, 1989.
39. Quinby WJ, Burke J, Trelstad R, *et al:* The use of microscopy as a guide to primary excision of high-tension electrical burns. *J Trauma* **18:** 423,1978.
40. Reilly JP: Scales of reaction to electric shock: thresholds and biophysical mechanisms. *Ann NY Acad Sci* **720:** 21-37, 1994.
41. Saffle JR, Davis B, Williams P, et al: Recent outcomes in the treatment of burn injury in the United States: A report from the American Burn Association Patient Registry. *J Burn Care Rehabil* **16:** 219-32,1995.
42. Tropea BI, Lee RC: Thermal injury kinetics in electrical trauma. *J Biomech Eng* **114:** 241-50,1992.
43. Tsong TY, Astumian RD: Electroconformational coupling and membrane protein function. *Prog Biophys Mol Biol* **50:**1-45, 1987.
44. Tung L, Tovar O, Neunlist M, Jain S, *et al:* Effects of strong electrical shock on cardiac muscle tissue. *Ann NY Acad Sci* **720:** 160-75, 1994.
45. Varghese G, Mani MM, Redford JB: Spinal cord injuries following electrical accidents. *Paraplegia* **24:** 159-66,1986.
46. Wilbourn AJ: Peripheral nerve disorders in electrical and lightning injuries. *Semin Neurol* **15:** 241-56,1995.
47. Zelt RG, Daniel RK, Ballard PA, *et al:* High-voltage electrical injuries': Chronic wound evaluation. *Plast Reconstr Surg* **82:** 1027-41, 1988.

Index